The DARK CALORIES cookbook

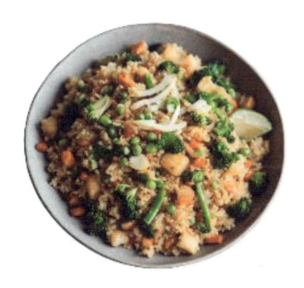

Harnessing the Power of Traditional Fats for Optimal Health and Flavor with Colorful Photos

Margaret Scott

Disclaimer Page

The information provided in this book is for educational and informational purposes only and is not intended as medical advice. The recipes and suggestions in this book are based on the author's research and personal experience. Before making any significant changes to your diet, it is recommended that you consult with a healthcare provider, nutritionist, or other qualified medical professional to determine what is appropriate for your individual health needs.

The author and publisher disclaim any liability arising directly or indirectly from the use or misuse of the information contained in this book. Every effort has been made to ensure the content is accurate and up-to-date as of the publication date.

However, the field of nutrition is constantly evolving, and new research may alter or change the recommendations provided herein. Individual results may vary. The success of the dietary and lifestyle changes suggested in this book may depend on various factors, including, but not limited to, individual health conditions, adherence to the program, and other external factors. This book is not a substitute for professional medical advice, diagnosis, or treatment.

Table of content

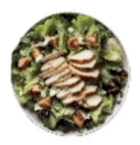

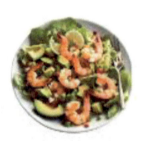

Introduction

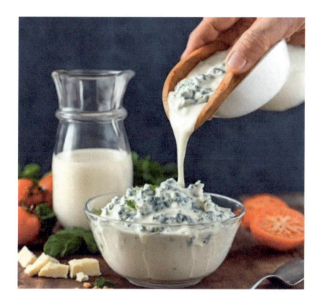

A few years ago, I found myself at a crossroads with my health. Despite following what I believed was a healthy diet; I was constantly battling fatigue, weight gain, and a general sense of unease. My meals were full of "heart-healthy" vegetable oils, low-fat products, and the latest super foods, yet I wasn't feeling super.

One day, while browsing research papers and books looking for answers, I stumbled upon a concept that changed my life: the idea that not all fats are created equal. It wasn't the butter or coconut oil in my diet that wreaked havoc on my health; it was the vegetable oils. Hidden in almost every processed food, these oils silently contributed to my declining health.

It was then that I discovered *"Dark Calories:"* The book resonated with me deeply, providing clear evidence that the very oils I had been told were beneficial were, in fact, anything but. The author's meticulous research and compelling arguments exposed the dangers lurking in these seemingly innocent oil bottles. I realized that I needed to change my kitchen radically if I wanted to reclaim my health.

My Journey to Health

Armed with this newfound knowledge, I began eliminating vegetable oils from my diet, replacing them with traditional fats like butter, Ghee, coconut, and olive oil. The transformation was nothing short of remarkable. Within weeks, I noticed a significant improvement in my energy levels, mental clarity, and weight. The chronic inflammation I had been experiencing began to subside, and I felt better than I had in years.

This personal journey inspired me to delve deeper into nutrition and cooking. I wanted to share this life-changing discovery with others, not just through facts and figures but through the meals that helped me heal. That's why I created this cookbook *The Dark Calories Cookbook* as a practical guide to help others experience the same benefits I did.

The Dark Side of Vegetable Oils

Vegetable oils, also known as seed oils, have become a staple in modern cooking. They are pervasive in our diets, found in everything from salad dressings to baked goods, fried foods, and snacks. However, their widespread use comes at a hidden cost. Unlike traditional fats that have nourished humans for centuries, vegetable oils are a relatively new addition to the human diet, introduced only in the last 150 years.

These highly processed oils, often extracted from genetically modified crops, are rich in omega-6 fatty acids. While omega-6 fatty acids are essential in small amounts, an excess can lead to chronic inflammation—a root cause of many modern diseases, including heart disease, diabetes, and cancer. The processing methods used to produce vegetable oils often involve high heat, chemical solvents, and deodorization, stripping the oils of their natural nutrients and creating harmful compounds like trans fats and free radicals.

Building on "Dark Calories"

If you've read "*Dark Calories:* you already know how these oils infiltrate our food supply and negatively impact our well-being. This cookbook is the next step—a practical companion to the original book. It offers a clear path to eliminating these oils from your diet and replacing them with healthful, traditional fats.

Rediscovering the Benefits of Traditional Fats

Traditional fats like butter, Ghee, coconut, and olive oil are minimally processed, nutrient-rich, and have a balanced fatty acid profile supporting optimal health. These fats have nourished humans for thousands of years, providing essential nutrients and stable energy without the harmful effects of vegetable oils.

Butter and Ghee, for example, are rich in butyrate, a short-chain fatty acid that supports gut health and reduces inflammation. Coconut oil contains medium-chain triglycerides (MCTs), which are quickly metabolized for energy and have been shown to support brain health and weight management. Olive oil, a staple of the Mediterranean diet, is packed with antioxidants and has been extensively studied for its heart-protective benefits.

How to Use This Cookbook

This cookbook is designed to help you transition away from harmful vegetable oils and embrace the rich, nourishing fats that have sustained human health for generations. Whether you're new to cooking with traditional fats or looking to expand your culinary repertoire, this book provides a variety of recipes that are as delicious as they are healthful.

In the following pages, you'll find 75 recipes divided into categories like breakfast, lunch, dinner, snacks, appetizers, sauces, and dressings. Each recipe is crafted to maximize flavor while ensuring only the best fats are used. From fluffy coconut flour pancakes to garlic butter steak and homemade olive oil dressings, these recipes will help you rediscover the joy of cooking with natural, wholesome ingredients.

The Journey Ahead

Changing from vegetable oils to traditional fats might seem daunting at first, but it can profoundly impact your health. This cookbook is not just about avoiding certain ingredients; it's about embracing a way of eating that nourishes your body from the inside out. By choosing the right fats, you'll not only improve your well-being but also contribute to the health of your loved ones.

As you explore these recipes, I encourage you to be mindful of your ingredients, where they come from, and how they affect your health. Cooking with traditional fats is more than a dietary choice; it's a return to time-honored practices prioritizing real food and natural health.

Let's embark on this journey together, one delicious meal at a time. Welcome to the **Dark Calories Cookbook**, where nourishing your body has never tasted so good.

Chapter 1

Overview of the Health Risks of Vegetable Oils

Vegetable oils, often promoted as heart-healthy alternatives, have become a staple in modern kitchens and processed foods. However, their widespread use is linked to various health risks frequently overlooked or misunderstood. These canola, soybean, corn, and sunflower oils are heavily processed and rich in omega-6 fatty acids. While omega-6 fatty acids are essential in small amounts, the excessive consumption typical in the modern diet creates an imbalance that promotes inflammation throughout the body.

1. Chronic Inflammation: The high levels of omega-6 fatty acids in vegetable oils can lead to an imbalance with omega-3 fatty acids, known for their anti-inflammatory properties. This imbalance is a significant contributor to chronic inflammation, a root cause of many modern diseases, including heart disease, diabetes, arthritis, and even certain types of cancer

2. Oxidative Stress: The processing methods used to extract vegetable oils often involve high heat and chemicals, which can create harmful byproducts such as free radicals. These free radicals cause oxidative stress in the body, damaging cells and DNA and accelerating aging.

3. Heart Disease: Contrary to the belief that vegetable oils are heart-healthy, studies have shown that they can increase the risk of heart disease. The high levels of omega-6 fatty acids can lead to the formation of arterial plaques, while the trans fats created during the processing of some vegetable oils have been directly linked to an increased risk of heart attacks and strokes.

4. Weight Gain and Obesity: Vegetable oils are calorie-dense and often found in processed foods that are easy to overconsume. Additionally, these oils can disrupt hormonal balance, leading to metabolism and fat storage issues, contributing to weight gain and obesity.

5. Insulin Resistance and Diabetes: Excessive vegetable oil consumption can cause chronic inflammation and oxidative stress, which can impair insulin function and lead to insulin resistance, a precursor to type 2 diabetes. The high omega-6 content also affects the body's ability to use glucose efficiently, increasing the risk of diabetes.

The Benefits of Traditional Fats

In contrast to vegetable oils, traditional fats have been a cornerstone of human diets for thousands of years. These fats, such as butter, Ghee, coconut, and olive oil, are minimally processed, nutrient-rich, and provide a balanced profile of fatty acids supporting overall health.

1. Stable at High Temperatures: Traditional fats like butter, Ghee, and coconut oil are stable at high temperatures, making them ideal for cooking. Unlike vegetable oils, which can oxidize and produce harmful compounds when heated, these fats maintain their nutritional integrity, reducing the risk of toxic byproducts.

2. Rich in Nutrients: Traditional fats are not just energy sources; they are also rich in fat-soluble vitamins and essential fatty acids. For example, butter and Ghee are excellent sources of vitamins A, D, E, and K, crucial for immune function, bone health, and skin health. Coconut oil contains medium-chain triglycerides (MCTs), which are quickly metabolized for energy and support brain health.

3. Anti-Inflammatory Properties: Unlike the inflammatory omega-6 fats in vegetable oils, traditional fats are either neutral or anti-inflammatory. Olive oil, a staple of the Mediterranean diet, is rich in monounsaturated fats and antioxidants, which have been shown to reduce inflammation and lower the risk of heart disease.

4. Supports Hormonal Health: Fats are essential for hormone production and balance. Traditional fats provide the building blocks for hormones, supporting everything from metabolism to reproductive health. For example, the cholesterol found in animal fats like butter and lard is necessary to produce vital hormones like estrogen and testosterone.

5. Improved Satiety and Weight Management: Traditional fats are satiating, meaning they help you feel full and satisfied after meals. This can lead to better portion control and reduced snacking, supporting weight management efforts. The stable energy these fats provide also prevents the blood sugar spikes and crashes familiar with high-carbohydrate, low-fat diets.

Key Ingredients and Tools for Cooking Without Vegetable Oils

Transitioning away from vegetable oils and embracing traditional fats requires a few simple adjustments in your kitchen. Here's what you'll need to get started:

Key Ingredients:

1. Butter and Ghee: Butter, especially from grass-fed cows, is rich in nutrients and flavor. Ghee, a clarified butter, is lactose-free and has a

higher smoke point, making it ideal for high-heat cooking.

2. Coconut Oil: Coconut oil is versatile and stable at high temperatures, making it perfect for frying, baking, and sautéing. It adds a subtle sweetness to dishes and is rich in MCTs.

3. Olive Oil: Extra virgin olive oil is best used for drizzling over salads, dipping bread, or finishing dishes. It's packed with antioxidants and heart-healthy monounsaturated fats.

4. Avocado Oil: Avocado oil has a high smoke point, making it excellent for grilling and roasting. It's also mild in flavor, so it won't overpower your dishes.

5. Animal Fats (Lard, Tallow, and Duck Fat): These traditional fats are perfect for roasting, frying, and adding depth to dishes. They are rich in flavor and nutrients, mainly when sourced from pasture-raised animals.

6. Full-Fat Dairy: Full-fat yogurt, cream, and cheese enrich dishes and provide essential nutrients like calcium and fat-soluble vitamins.

Essential Tools

1. Cast Iron Skillet: A cast iron skillet retains heat well and is perfect for high-heat cooking with traditional fats. It also adds a natural source of iron to your meals.

2. Stainless Steel or Ceramic Pans: These pans are ideal for cooking without the risk of harmful non-stick coatings leaching into your food. They work well with fats like butter, Ghee, and coconut oil.

3. Glass Storage Containers: Store your homemade dressings, sauces, and prepped ingredients in glass containers to avoid chemicals found in plastic.

4. Oil Dispensers: Invest in good-quality oil dispensers for your olive oil and avocado oil. This makes it easier to control portions and keep your oils fresh.

5. High-Quality Knives: Sharp, high-quality knives make preparing whole foods more accessible and more enjoyable. They're essential for chopping vegetables, slicing meats, and more.

By stocking your kitchen with these ingredients and tools, you'll be well-equipped to cook delicious, nourishing meals without relying on harmful vegetable oils. Embracing traditional fats in your cooking enhances the flavor and texture of your dishes and supports your long-term health.

Cooking Tips and Techniques

Transitioning away from vegetable oils and incorporating traditional fats into your diet can be a rewarding journey toward better health. However, it can also be daunting if you're accustomed to using vegetable oils in everyday cooking. This chapter provides practical tips and techniques to help you make this transition smoothly, store and use traditional fats effectively, and ensure that you're getting the most out of your ingredients.

How to Transition Away from Vegetable Oils

Switching from vegetable oils to traditional fats requires a mindset shift and a few adjustments in your cooking routine. Here are some strategies to help you make the transition:

1. Start Small: Begin by replacing vegetable oils in your most frequently used recipes. For example, swap canola or sunflower oil with olive oil in your salad dressings, or use butter or Ghee instead of margarine to spread on toast or baking.

2. Identify Hidden Sources of Vegetable Oils: Vegetable oils, including sauces, dressings, baked goods, and snacks, are often hidden in processed foods. Start reading labels more carefully and choose products that use traditional fats or, better yet, make your own from scratch.

3. Experiment with Different Fats: Each traditional fat has its own unique flavor and cooking properties. Experiment with different fats in your recipes to discover which ones you prefer for various dishes. For example, coconut oil adds a sweet, tropical flavor, while Ghee offers a rich, nutty taste.

4. Cook at Home More Often: Cooking at home gives you complete control over the fats you use. Dining out often means exposure to vegetable oils, so cooking at home ensures you stick to your commitment to avoid them.

5. Replace One Meal at a Time: Focus on one meal at a time—start with breakfast, then move on to lunch, and finally dinner. This gradual approach makes the transition feel more manageable and sustainable.

6. Learn to Make Homemade Versions: Many store-bought products contain vegetable oils, like mayonnaise, salad dressings, and baked goods. Learn to make these items at home using traditional fats. Not only will this help you avoid vegetable oils, but it will also improve the taste and quality of your meals.

7. Plan Ahead: Keep your pantry stocked with traditional fats and ingredients, so you're always prepared to cook meals without using vegetable oils. Planning your meals can also help you avoid the temptation of convenience foods that contain vegetable oils.

8. Educate Yourself: The more you understand the benefits of traditional fats and the risks of vegetable oils, the more motivated you'll be to stick with the change. Continue reading, researching, and learning about the impact of fats on your health.

The Best Ways to Store and Use Traditional Fats

Proper storage and usage of traditional fats are essential to maintain their quality and ensure they remain fresh and practical in your cooking. Here's how to handle different types of fats:

1. Butter and Ghee

Storage

Butter can be stored in the refrigerator for up to two months or in the freezer for up to six months. Due to its lack of water content, Ghee is more stable and can be stored at room temperature in a cool, dark place for up to six months or in the refrigerator for even longer.

Usage

Butter is excellent for baking, sautéing, and adding richness to dishes. With its higher smoke point, Ghee is ideal for frying, roasting, and high-heat cooking. Both add a delicious, creamy flavor to your meals.

2. Coconut Oil:

Storage

Coconut oil is solid at room temperature and can be stored in a pantry for up to two years. Please keep it in a cool, dark place away from direct sunlight.

Usage

Coconut oil is versatile and can be used for frying, baking, and sautéing. It works well in sweet and savory dishes and adds a mild coconut flavor, enhancing tropical and Asian-inspired recipes.

3. Olive Oil

Storage

Extra virgin olive oil should be stored in a cool, dark place away from heat and light. If unopened, it can last up to two years, but once opened, it's best used within six months to a year for optimal flavor and nutritional value.

Usage

Olive oil is perfect for drizzling over salads, dipping bread, and finishing dishes. While it can be used for cooking, it's best for low to medium-heat applications to preserve its delicate flavors and nutrients.

4. Avocado Oil:

Storage

Avocado oil should be stored in a cool, dark place, much like olive oil. Its shelf life is about one year if unopened, and once opened, it should be used within six months.

- ### Usage:

Avocado oil has a high smoke point, making it excellent for frying, grilling, and roasting. Its mild flavor makes it versatile for various dishes, from dressings to marinades

Storage

Store rendered animal fats in the refrigerator for up to six months or in the freezer for up to a year. These fats are stable and don't quickly go rancid, but keeping them cool extends their shelf life.

These fats are ideal for roasting, frying, and adding depth to savory dishes. They impart a rich, umami flavor for hearty meals like stews and roasts.

Sourcing Quality Ingredients

The quality of the fats you use in cooking is just as important as the type of fat. Here are some tips for sourcing the best ingredients:

1. Choose Organic and Grass-Fed: Whenever possible, choose organic butter and Ghee from grass-fed cows. Grass-fed butter is higher in nutrients like vitamin K2 and conjugated linoleic acid (CLA), which have anti-inflammatory and heart-protective properties.

2. Cold-Pressed and Unrefined Oils: Look for cold-pressed and unrefined versions of oils like coconut and olive oil. These oils are processed at lower temperatures, preserving their nutritional content and natural flavor.

3. Local and Sustainable Sources: Sourcing your fats from local and sustainable farms supports regional agriculture and ensures that the animals are raised humanely, leading to higher-quality products. Visit local farmers' markets or look for trusted suppliers online.

Ghee or tallow can enhance the flavor and richness of the dish.

4. Grilling: Grilling is another great way to cook meats and vegetables while retaining nutrients. To

4. Check for Purity: Ensure that the oils and fats you buy are 100% pure and not mixed with other, lower-quality oils. For example, some olive oils are diluted with cheaper vegetable oils, so checking the label and buying from reputable brands is essential.

5. Buy in Bulk and Store Properly: Purchasing in bulk can be more cost-effective, especially for items like coconut oil and Ghee. Just be sure to store them properly to maintain their freshness over time.

Cooking Methods that Retain Nutrients

How you cook your food can impact the nutrient content of your meals. Here are some cooking methods that help retain the nutritional value of your ingredients while using traditional fats:

1. Sautéing and Stir-Frying: Sautéing vegetables and proteins in traditional fats like butter, Ghee, or coconut oil is a quick and efficient way to retain their nutrients. The high heat and short cooking time minimize nutrient loss.

2. Roasting: Roasting meats and vegetables in animal fats or avocado oil helps lock in moisture and flavor. This method caramelizes the natural sugars in vegetables, enhancing their sweetness and nutritional profile.

3. Slow Cooking: Slow cooking at low temperatures, especially with fatty cuts of meat, allows for nutrient retention and makes the proteins more digestible. Adding a healthy fat like

keep your meats moist and flavorful, baste them with a traditional fat like olive oil or butter.

5. Baking: Baking with traditional fats like butter or coconut oil improves the texture and taste of baked goods and adds nutritional value. Use these fats to replace vegetable oils in recipes for a healthier outcome.

6. Blanching and Steaming: Blanching or steaming vegetables is a gentle cooking method that helps retain vitamins and minerals. After blanching or boiling, toss the vegetables in butter or olive oil for added flavor and nutrients.

Chapter 2

Breakfast recipes

Why Breakfast Matters

Breakfast is often hailed as the most important meal of the day, and for good reason. After a night of fasting, your body needs nourishment to kick start your metabolism, provide energy for the day ahead, and stabilize your blood sugar levels. A well-balanced breakfast sets the tone for how you'll feel and perform throughout the day, influencing everything from your mood to your cognitive function.

However, the typical modern breakfast often loaded with refined carbohydrates, sugars, and unhealthy fats can do more harm than good. Instead of providing sustained energy, these foods can lead to spikes and blood sugar crashes, leaving you tired and hungry shortly after eating. That's why choosing the right ingredients, particularly the fats you use, is crucial to building a breakfast that truly supports your health.

Choosing the Right Fats for a Healthy Start

The fats you include in your breakfast can significantly affect how you feel throughout the day. Traditional fats, such as butter, ghee, coconut, and olive oil, provide a steady energy source, help you feel full longer, and support your body's essential functions. These nutrient-dense fats offer fat-soluble vitamins and essential fatty acids that your body needs to function optimally.

Butter and Ghee

Starting your day with butter or ghee, mainly when sourced from grass-fed cows, provides your body with vitamins A, D, E, and K2 and conjugated linoleic acid (CLA), which has anti-inflammatory properties. These fats are also rich in butyrate, a short-chain fatty acid that supports gut health.

Coconut Oil

Coconut oil is another excellent choice for breakfast, mainly because of its medium-chain triglycerides (MCTs). MCTs are rapidly absorbed and converted into energy, making coconut oil an ideal fat for those looking to boost their metabolism and maintain energy levels throughout the morning.

Olive Oil

Extra virgin olive oil, a staple of the Mediterranean diet, is rich in monounsaturated fats and antioxidants. It's a heart-healthy fat that can be drizzled over eggs, used in dressings for morning salads, or incorporated into savory breakfast dishes.

Avocado Oil

Avocado oil is another versatile fat that's mild in flavor and high in monounsaturated fats. It's great for cooking at higher temperatures and adds a subtle, creamy texture to dishes.

By incorporating these traditional fats into your breakfast, you'll set yourself up for a day of sustained energy, improved focus, and better overall health. Now, let's dive into the recipes to help you make the most of these nourishing fats.

Classic Scrambled Eggs with Grass-Fed Butter

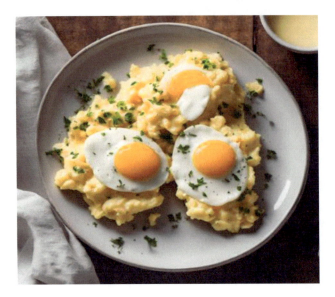

Scrambled eggs are a breakfast staple enjoyed around the world, but what sets this version apart is the use of grass-fed butter. Unlike conventional butter, grass-fed butter provides a creamier, richer flavor that elevates this simple dish to a gourmet experience.

Ingredients

- 4 large eggs (preferably organic and pasture-raised)
- 2 tablespoons grass-fed butter
- Salt and pepper to taste
- Fresh herbs (such as chives or parsley) for garnish (optional)

Instructions

1. Whisk the Eggs: Crack the eggs into a bowl and whisk them until the yolks and whites are thoroughly combined. Whisking introduces air, which helps to make the eggs fluffy.

2. Prepare the Pan: Heat a non-stick skillet over low to medium heat. Add the grass-fed butter to the pan and let it melt slowly. The butter should foam but not brown, ensuring it retains its rich flavor without becoming bitter.

3. Cook the Eggs: Pour the whisked eggs into the skillet. Let them sit undisturbed for a few seconds to begin setting at the bottom. Then, gently stir with a spatula, bringing the cooked edges towards the center. Continue to stir gently, allowing the eggs to cook evenly.

4. Season and Serve: Remove the pan from the heat before the eggs are fully set. The residual heat will finish cooking the eggs, keeping them soft and creamy season with salt and pepper to taste. Garnish with fresh herbs if desired.

5. Plate and Enjoy: Serve immediately for the best texture. Pair with whole-grain toast or fresh fruit for a complete, nourishing breakfast.

Chef's Tips

- **Low and Slow:** Cooking the eggs over low heat ensures they stay tender and creamy. High heat can make the eggs rubbery and overcooked.
- **Butter's Role:** Using grass-fed butter adds flavor and helps achieve the perfect creamy texture. Add a small pat of butter just before serving for an extra-rich taste.

Nutritional Information

Calories: 300 | Protein: 14g | Total Fat: 27g | Saturated Fat: 15g | Cholesterol: 372mg | Sodium: 220mg | Fiber: 0g | Vitamin A: 15% DV | Vitamin D: 20% DV | Vitamin K2: High (due to grass-fed butter)

Serving

- **With Toast:** Serve alongside a slice of sourdough or whole-grain toast to soak up the rich, buttery eggs.

- **As a Wrap:** Roll the scrambled eggs in a whole-grain tortilla with some sautéed vegetables for a portable breakfast option

Coconut Flour Pancakes with Pure Maple Syrup

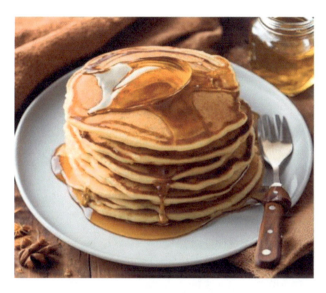

These light and fluffy pancakes are made with coconut flour, offering a deliciously gluten-free option for breakfast. Coconut flour is fiber-rich, giving these pancakes a subtle, natural sweetness that pairs perfectly with pure maple syrup.

Ingredients

- 1/4 cup coconut flour
- 1/4 teaspoon baking powder
- 4 large eggs
- 1/4 cup full-fat coconut milk
- 1 tablespoon coconut oil, melted
- 1 teaspoon vanilla extract
- Coconut oil for cooking
- Pure maple syrup for serving

Instructions

1. Mix the Dry Ingredients: Combine the coconut flour and baking powder in a mixing bowl.

2. Add the Wet Ingredients: Add the eggs, coconut milk, melted coconut oil, and vanilla extract to the dry ingredients. Mix until the batter is smooth.

3. Cook the Pancakes: Heat a small amount of coconut oil in a non-stick skillet over medium heat. Pour batter into the skillet to form small pancakes. Cook until bubbles form on the surface, then flip and cook until golden brown.

4. Serve: Serve warm with a drizzle of pure maple syrup.

Chef's Tips

- **Thickness Control:** Add more coconut milk to reach your desired consistency if the batter is too thick.

- **Cooking Tip:** Cook the pancakes on medium heat to ensure they cook through without burning.

Nutritional Information

Calories: 250 | Protein: 10g | Total Fat: 20g | Saturated Fat: 14g | Cholesterol: 220mg | Sodium: 140mg | Fiber: 6g | Vitamin D: 8% DV

Serving

- **With Fresh Berries:** Top with fresh berries for extra flavor and nutrients.

- **With Nuts:** Sprinkle with chopped nuts for added crunch and healthy fats.

Avocado and Poached Egg Toast on Sourdough

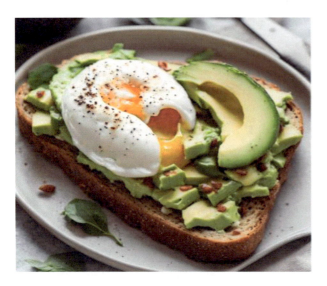

This dish combines the creamy richness of avocado with a perfectly poached egg atop toasted sourdough bread. It's a simple yet satisfying breakfast packed with healthy fats and protein.

Ingredients

- 1 ripe avocado
- 2 slices sourdough bread
- 2 large eggs
- 1 tablespoon extra-virgin olive oil
- Salt and pepper to taste
- Red pepper flakes (optional, for garnish)

Instructions

1. Toast the Bread: Toast the sourdough bread slices until golden brown.

2. Prepare the Avocado: Mash the avocado and spread it evenly on the toasted bread season with salt and pepper.

3. Poach the Eggs: Poach the eggs in simmering water until the whites are set but the yolks remain runny.

4. Assemble: Place the poached eggs on top of the avocado toast. Drizzle with olive oil and sprinkle with red pepper flakes if desired.

Chef's Tips

- **Perfect Poaching:** Add a tablespoon of vinegar to the simmering water to help the egg whites set quickly and keep their shape.

- **Extra Flavor:** Rub a garlic clove on the toast before adding the avocado for an additional layer of flavor.

Nutritional Information

Calories: 350 | Protein: 12g | Total Fat: 28g | Saturated Fat: 5g | Cholesterol: 190mg | Sodium: 320mg | Fiber: 8g | Vitamin E: 15% DV

Serving

- **With Greens:** Serve with a side of mixed greens or arugula for a fresh and light addition.

- **As a Sandwich:** For a heartier meal, top with an extra slice of toasted sourdough and serve as an open-faced sandwich.

Full-fat Greek Yogurt with Berries and Honey

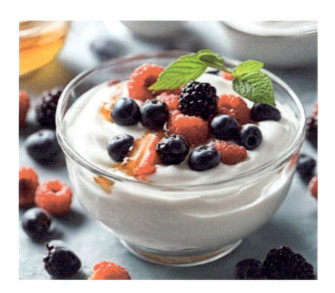

This simple and refreshing breakfast pairs the creaminess of full-fat Greek yogurt with the natural sweetness of fresh berries and honey. It's a quick, nutritious option that's perfect for busy mornings.

Ingredients

- 1 cup full-fat Greek yogurt
- 1/2 cup mixed fresh berries (strawberries, blueberries, raspberries)
- 1 tablespoon raw honey
- 1 tablespoon chopped nuts or granola (optional)

Instructions

1. Prepare the Yogurt: Scoop the Greek yogurt into a bowl.

2. Add the Berries: Top the yogurt with the mixed fresh berries.

3. Drizzle with Honey: Drizzle the honey over the berries and yogurt.

4. Serve: Add chopped nuts or granola on top if desired for extra texture and crunch.

Chef's Tips:

- **Yogurt Choice:** Choose full-fat Greek yogurt for its rich flavor and creamier texture, providing more satiety.
- **Honey Substitute:** If you prefer less sweetness, you can replace the honey with a sprinkle of cinnamon.

Nutritional Information

Calories: 250 | Protein: 10g | Total Fat: 12g | Saturated Fat: 7g | Cholesterol: 35mg | Sodium: 50mg | Fiber: 4g | Calcium: 20% DV

Serving

- **With Seeds:** Sprinkle chia seeds or flaxseeds on top for added fiber and omega-3s.
- **On-the-Go:** Layer the ingredients in a mason jar for a portable breakfast option.

Almond Flour Waffles with Ghee

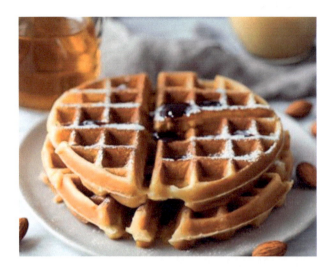

These almond flour waffles are a delicious grain-free alternative to traditional waffles. Cooking them in ghee adds a rich, nutty flavor while keeping the waffles crisp on the outside and soft on the inside.

Ingredients

- 1 1/2 cups almond flour
- 1/4 teaspoon baking soda
- 2 large eggs
- 1/4 cup full-fat coconut milk
- 2 tablespoons ghee, melted
- 1 teaspoon vanilla extract
- Ghee for cooking

Instructions

1. Mix the Dry Ingredients: Combine almond flour and baking soda in a mixing bowl.

2. Add the Wet Ingredients: Stir in the eggs, coconut milk, melted ghee, and vanilla extract until the batter is smooth.

3. Cook the Waffles: Preheat a waffle iron and grease it with ghee. Pour the batter into the waffle iron and cook until the waffles are golden brown and crisp.

4. Serve: Serve the waffles warm with additional ghee, fresh fruit, or a drizzle of maple syrup.

Chef's Tips

- **Crispy Waffles:** Leave extra crispy waffles in the waffle iron for a bit longer after they turn golden brown.

- **Freezing Option:** These waffles freeze well; reheat them in a toaster or oven for a quick breakfast.

Nutritional Information

Calories: 320 | Protein: 10g | Total Fat: 28g | Saturated Fat: 10g | Cholesterol: 140mg | Sodium: 120mg | Fiber: 4g | Magnesium: 15% dv

Serving

- **With Fruit:** Mix fresh berries or banana slices for a naturally sweet addition.

- **With Whipped Cream:** Add a dollop of whipped coconut cream or full-fat cream for a decadent treats.

Chia Seed Pudding with Coconut Milk

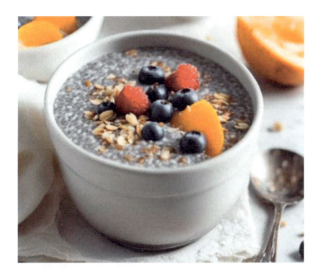

Chia seed pudding is a versatile and nutrient-dense breakfast that's easy to prepare in advance. The chia seeds absorb the coconut milk, creating a creamy, pudding-like texture perfect for layering with fruits and nuts.

Ingredients

- 1/4 cup chia seeds
- 1 cup full-fat coconut milk
- 1 teaspoon vanilla extract
- 1 tablespoon maple syrup or honey (optional)
- Fresh fruit or nuts for topping

Instructions

1. Combine the Ingredients: In a mixing bowl, whisk together the chia seeds, coconut milk, vanilla extract, and sweetener if using.

2. Refrigerate: Cover the bowl and refrigerate for at least 4 hours or overnight, allowing the chia seeds to absorb the liquid and thicken into a pudding.

3. Serve: Stir the pudding and serve it with fresh fruit or nuts.

Chef's Tips

- **Consistency Check:** If the pudding is too thick after chilling, stir in more coconut milk until you reach your desired consistency.

- **Flavor Variations:** Add cocoa powder for a chocolate version or matcha powder for a green tea twist.

Nutritional Information

Calories: 250 | Protein: 5g | Total Fat: 20g | Saturated Fat: 14g | Cholesterol: 0mg | Sodium: 15mg | Fiber: 10g | Omega-3s: High

Serving

- **With Berries:** Top with fresh berries like strawberries or blueberries for added flavor and antioxidants.

- **As a Parfait:** Layer the chia pudding with granola and yogurt in a glass for a visually appealing parfait.

Smoked Salmon and Cream Cheese Omelette

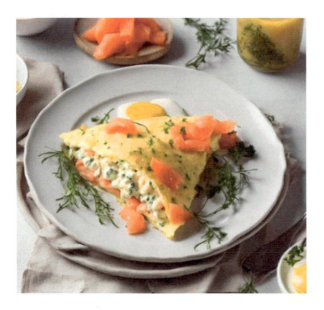

This luxurious omelet combines the rich flavors of smoked salmon with the creaminess of softened cream cheese. It's a satisfying breakfast for a memorable morning or a quick weekday treat.

Ingredients

- 3 large eggs
- 2 ounces smoked salmon, sliced
- 2 tablespoons cream cheese, softened
- 1 tablespoon butter (preferably grass-fed)
- 1 tablespoon fresh dill, chopped (optional)
- Salt and pepper to taste

Instructions

1. **Whisk the Eggs:** In a bowl, whisk the eggs until well combined and slightly frothy.

2. **Prepare the Pan:** Heat the butter in a non-stick skillet over medium heat until melted and bubbling.

3. **Cook the Omelette:** Pour the eggs into the skillet. Cook without stirring until the edges begin to set. Gently lift the edges with a spatula, allowing the uncooked eggs to flow underneath.

4. **Add Fillings:** Once the eggs are mostly set, place the smoked salmon and dollops of cream cheese on one half of the omelet—season with salt and pepper.

5. **Fold and Serve:** Fold the omelet in half and cook for another minute until the cheese is warmed. Slide the omelet onto a plate and garnish with fresh dill if desired.

Chef's Tips

- **Even Cooking:** Keep the heat medium to avoid overcooking the eggs and maintain a soft texture.

- **Cream Cheese:** Soften the cream cheese before adding it to the omelet for easier spreading.

Nutritional Information

Calories: 350 | Protein: 20g | Total Fat: 30g | Saturated Fat: 12g | Cholesterol: 410mg | Sodium: 600mg | Omega-3s: High

Serving

- **With Greens:** Serve with mixed greens lightly dressed with olive oil and lemon juice for a fresh, light contrast.

- **With Whole-Grain Toast:** Pair with a slice of whole-grain toast for added texture and fiber.

Spinach and Feta Frittata

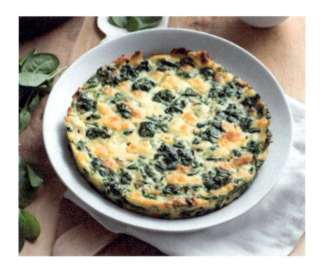

This spinach and feta frittata is a simple yet flavorful dish perfect for a weekend brunch or a make-ahead breakfast. The salty feta complements the earthiness of the spinach, creating a well-balanced meal.

Ingredients

- 6 large eggs
- 1 cup fresh spinach, chopped
- 1/2 cup feta cheese, crumbled
- 1/4 cup milk or cream
- 1 tablespoon olive oil
- 1 clove garlic, minced
- Salt and pepper to taste

Instructions

1. **Preheat the Oven:** Preheat your oven to 375°F (190°C).

2. **Sauté the Spinach:** Heat the olive oil in an oven-safe skillet over medium heat. Add the garlic and cook until fragrant. Add the spinach and sauté until wilted.

3. **Prepare the Egg Mixture:** In a bowl, whisk together the eggs, milk or cream, salt, and pepper. Stir in the crumbled feta.

4. **Combine and Cook:** Pour the egg mixture over the sautéed spinach in the skillet. Stir gently to combine. Cook on the stovetop for 2-3 minutes until the edges start to set.

5. **Bake:** Transfer the skillet to the preheated oven and bake for 10-12 minutes, or until the frittata is fully set and slightly golden on top.

6. **Serve:** Allow the frittata to cool slightly before slicing and serving.

Chef's Tips

- **Customizable:** Add other vegetables like bell peppers or onions to the frittata for more variety.

- **Cheese Substitution:** Substitute feta with goat cheese or shredded mozzarella for a milder flavor.

Nutritional Information

Calories: 280 | Protein: 18g | Total Fat: 20g | Saturated Fat: 8g | Cholesterol: 350mg | Sodium: 450mg | Fiber: 2g

Serving

- **With Salad:** Serve with a side salad of mixed greens, tomatoes, and cucumbers dressed in lemon and olive oil.

- **As Leftovers:** Frittata slices can be stored in the refrigerator and enjoyed cold or reheated for a quick meal.

Bulletproof Coffee with MCT Oil

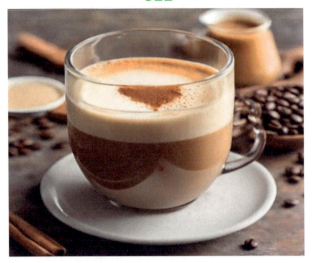

Bulletproof coffee is a high-fat, low-carb drink that has gained popularity in ketogenic and low-carb communities. Made with quality coffee, MCT oil, and butter, it provides a quick, energy-boosting breakfast option that keeps you full for hours.

Ingredients

- 1 cup brewed coffee (preferably organic)
- 1 tablespoon MCT oil
- 1 tablespoon unsalted grass-fed butter or ghee

Instructions

1. **Brew the Coffee:** Brew a fresh coffee using your preferred method.
2. **Blend the Ingredients:** In a blender, combine the hot coffee, MCT oil, and butter. Blend on high for 20-30 seconds until frothy.
3. **Serve:** Pour into a mug and enjoy immediately.

Chef's Tips

- **Blending Tip:** Blending the coffee ensures the fats emulsify correctly, creating a creamy, latte-like texture.
- **Sweetening:** If you prefer a sweeter coffee, add a touch of stevia or a teaspoon of vanilla extract.

Nutritional Information:

Calories: 220 | Protein: 0g | Total Fat: 24g | Saturated Fat: 14g | Cholesterol: 30mg | Sodium: 20mg | Carbohydrates: 0g

Serving

- **With Collagen:** Add a scoop of collagen powder for an extra protein boost and health benefits.
- **As a Meal Replacement:** Bulletproof coffee is often used as a meal replacement for breakfast, particularly in low-carb diets.

Bacon and Egg Muffins

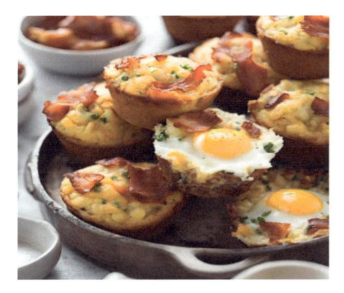

These bacon and egg muffins are a portable, protein-packed breakfast option for busy mornings. Crispy bacon and fluffy eggs combine to create a satisfying, low-carb meal that can be made ahead of time.

Ingredients

- 6 large eggs
- 6 slices bacon
- 1/4 cup cheddar cheese, shredded
- 1/4 cup bell peppers, diced
- Salt and pepper to taste
- Fresh parsley, chopped (optional)

Instructions

1. **Preheat the Oven:** Preheat your oven to 350°F (175°C).

2. **Cook the Bacon:** Cook the bacon in a skillet until crispy. Remove it and drain on paper towels, then chop it into bite-sized pieces.

3. **Prepare the Egg Mixture:** Whisk the eggs in a bowl and season with salt and pepper. Stir in the cheddar cheese and diced bell peppers.

4. **Assemble the Muffins:** Grease a muffin tin with cooking spray or butter. Divide the chopped bacon among the muffin cups, and then pour the egg mixture over the bacon.

5. **Bake:** Bake for 15-20 minutes until the eggs are fully set and slightly golden on top.

6. **Serve:** Allow the muffins to cool slightly before removing them from the tin. If desired, garnish with fresh parsley.

Chef's Tips

- **Make-Ahead:** These muffins can be made in advance and stored in the refrigerator for up to 5 days. Reheat them in the microwave or oven before serving.

- **Vegetable Options:** Feel free to add other vegetables like spinach or mushrooms for more flavor and nutrition.

Nutritional Information

Calories: 180 | Protein: 12g | Total Fat: 14g | Saturated Fat: 6g | Cholesterol: 220mg | Sodium: 400mg | Fiber: 0g

Serving

- **On-the-Go:** These muffins are perfect for a grab-and-go breakfast. Pair with a piece of fruit for a balanced meal.

- **With Avocado:** Serve alongside sliced avocado for added healthy fats and creaminess.

Sweet Potato Hash with Eggs and Avocado Oil

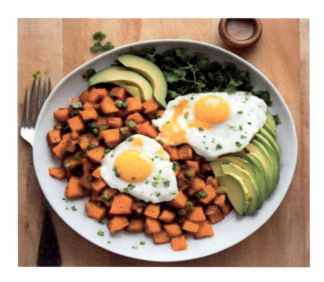

This sweet potato hash is a hearty and nutritious breakfast dish. It features crispy sweet potatoes, savory spices, and perfectly cooked eggs. Cooking with avocado oil adds a subtle flavor and ensures a high smoke point for crisping the potatoes.

Ingredients

- 2 medium sweet potatoes, peeled and diced
- 1 small onion, diced
- 1 red bell pepper, diced
- 2 tablespoons avocado oil
- 1 teaspoon smoked paprika
- Salt and pepper to taste
- 4 large eggs

Instructions

1. Cook the Vegetables: Heat the avocado oil in a large skillet over medium heat. Add the sweet potatoes, onion, and bell pepper. Season with smoked paprika, salt, and pepper. Cook, stirring occasionally, until the sweet potatoes are tender and slightly crispy.

2. Create Space for Eggs: Once the vegetables are cooked, create four small wells in the hash and crack an egg into each well.

3. Cook the Eggs: Cover the skillet and cook until the eggs reach your desired level of doneness, with firm whites and runny or set yolks.

4. Serve: Serve the hash immediately, either as is or with a drizzle of hot sauce for extra flavor.

Chef's Tips

- **Even Cooking:** Cut the sweet potatoes into small, even cubes to ensure they cook through evenly.

- **Spice It Up:** Add a pinch of cayenne pepper or chili flakes for some heat.

Nutritional Information

Calories: 350 | Protein: 12g | Total Fat: 18g | Saturated Fat: 4g | Cholesterol: 190mg | Sodium: 220mg | Fiber: 6g

Serving:

- **With Avocado:** Serve with sliced avocado for added creaminess and healthy fats.

- **As a Side:** Pair with a green salad or sautéed greens for a complete meal.

Keto-Friendly Smoothie with Coconut Milk

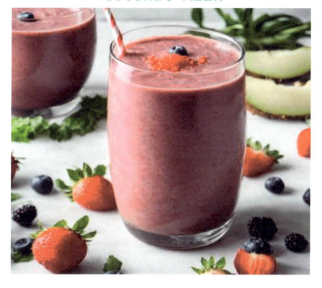

This keto-friendly smoothie is rich, creamy, and packed with healthy fats from coconut milk and avocado. It's a perfect low-carb breakfast or snack that keeps you full and energized.

Ingredients

- 1/2 avocado

- 1/2 cup full-fat coconut milk

- 1/2 cup water or unsweetened almond milk

- 1 tablespoon MCT oil or coconut oil

- 1/2 cup spinach leaves

- 1/4 teaspoon vanilla extract

- 1-2 drops liquid stevia (optional)

- Ice cubes (optional)

Instructions

1. Combine Ingredients: In a blender, combine the avocado, coconut milk, water or almond milk, MCT oil, spinach, vanilla extract, and stevia.

2, Blend: Blend on high until the mixture is smooth and creamy. Add ice cubes if you prefer a colder, thicker smoothie.

3. Serve: Pour into a glass and enjoy immediately.

Chef's Tips

- **Customize:** Add a scoop of collagen powder or protein powder for extra protein.

- **Sweetness Level:** Adjust the sweetness by adding more or less stevia, or omit it entirely if you prefer.

Nutritional Information

Calories: 300 | Protein: 2g | Total Fat: 30g | Saturated Fat: 22g | Cholesterol: 0mg | Sodium: 40mg | Fiber: 6g

Serving

- **With Seeds:** Sprinkle chia seeds or flaxseeds on top for added texture and fiber.

- **As a Bowl:** Turn this smoothie into a smoothie bowl by reducing the liquid and topping it with nuts, seeds, and berries.

Grain-Free Granola with Nuts and Seeds

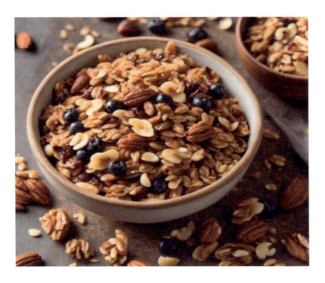

This grain-free granola is a crunchy, satisfying alternative to traditional granola, made with a blend of nuts, seeds, and coconut flakes. It's lightly sweetened with honey and flavored with warm spices, making it perfect for a healthy breakfast or snack.

Ingredients

- 1 cup raw almonds, chopped
- 1 cup raw walnuts, chopped
- 1/2 cup raw pumpkin seeds (pepitas)
- 1/2 cup raw sunflower seeds
- 1/2 cup unsweetened coconut flakes
- 1/4 cup chia seeds
- 2 tablespoons flaxseeds
- 1/4 cup coconut oil, melted
- 1/4 cup raw honey or maple syrup
- 1 teaspoon vanilla extract
- 1 teaspoon cinnamon
- 1/4 teaspoon salt

Instructions

1. Preheat the Oven: Preheat your oven to 300°F (150°C) and line a baking sheet with parchment paper.

2. **Mix the Dry Ingredients:** In a large mixing bowl, combine the almonds, walnuts, pumpkin seeds, sunflower seeds, coconut flakes, chia seeds, and flaxseeds.

3. **Prepare the Wet Mixture:** In a separate bowl, whisk together the melted coconut oil, honey or maple syrup, vanilla extract, cinnamon, and salt.

4. **Combine and Bake:** Pour the wet mixture over the dry ingredients and stir until everything is well coated. Spread the mixture evenly on the prepared baking sheet.

5. **Bake:** Bake for 20-25 minutes, stirring halfway through, until the granola is golden brown and fragrant.

6. **Cool and Store:** Allow the granola to cool completely on the baking sheet. Once cooled, store in an airtight container at room temperature for up to two weeks.

Chef's Tips

- **Customization:** Feel free to mix and match your favorite nuts and seeds. You can also add dried fruit after baking for additional sweetness.

- **Serving:** Serve with full-fat yogurt, almond milk, or as a topping for smoothie bowls.

Nutritional Information

Calories: 200 (per 1/4 cup serving) | Protein: 5g | Total Fat: 18g | Saturated Fat: 6g | Cholesterol: 0mg | Sodium: 40mg | Fiber: 4g

Serving

- **With Yogurt:** Serve over full-fat Greek yogurt with fresh berries for a balanced breakfast.

- **As a Snack:** Enjoy it by the handful as a crunchy, satisfying snack throughout the day.

Shakshuka with Olive Oil

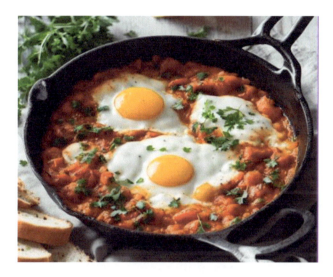

Shakshuka is a North African and Middle Eastern dish of poached eggs in a spicy tomato and pepper sauce. It is hearty and flavorful and perfect for breakfast, brunch, or dinner. Cooking it in high-quality olive oil enhances the rich flavors and adds a depth of nutrition.

Ingredients

- 2 tablespoons extra virgin olive oil

- 1 onion, diced

- 1 red bell pepper, diced

- 3 cloves garlic, minced

- 1 teaspoon ground cumin

- 1 teaspoon smoked paprika

- 1/4 teaspoon cayenne pepper (optional)

- 1 can (14.5 ounces) diced tomatoes

- Salt and pepper to taste

- 4-6 large eggs

- Fresh cilantro or parsley, chopped (for garnish)

Instructions

1. **Sauté the Vegetables:** Heat the olive oil in a large skillet over medium heat. Add the diced onion and bell pepper, and cook until softened about 5-7 minutes. Stir in the garlic, cumin, smoked paprika, and cayenne pepper, and cook for an additional minute until fragrant.

2. **Add the Tomatoes:** Pour in the diced tomatoes (with their juices) and season with salt and pepper. Reduce the heat to low and let the sauce simmer for 10-15 minutes until slightly thickened.

3. **Poach the Eggs:** Using the back of a spoon, make small wells in the sauce and crack an egg into each well. Cover the skillet and cook for 5-7 minutes or until the eggs are set to your desired doneness.

4. **Garnish and Serve:** Remove the skillet from the heat and garnish with fresh cilantro or parsley. Serve immediately with crusty bread or as is.

Chef's Tips

- **Spice Level:** Adjust the spice level by adding more or less cayenne pepper to the sauce.

- **Cooking Tip:** For a richer flavor, cook the sauce longer to allow the flavors to meld together before adding the eggs.

Nutritional Information

Serving

- **With Bread:** Serve with crusty bread or pita to dip into the flavorful sauce.

- **As a Main Course,** Pair it with a simple green salad for a complete meal.

Coconut Flour Breakfast Biscuits

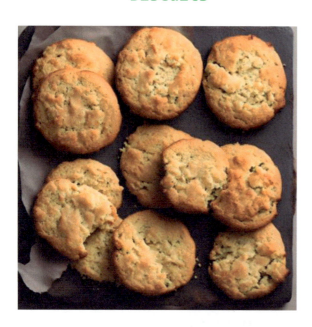

These coconut flour biscuits are a delightful grain-free option for breakfast. They're light, fluffy, and slightly sweet, perfect for serving with butter, honey, or your favorite jam.

Ingredients

- 1/2 cup coconut flour
- 1/2 teaspoon baking soda
- 1/4 teaspoon salt
- 4 large eggs
- 1/4 cup coconut oil, melted
- 1 tablespoon honey or maple syrup (optional)
- 1/2 teaspoon apple cider vinegar

Instructions

1. **Preheat the Oven:** Preheat your oven to 350°F (175°C) and line a baking sheet with parchment paper.

2. **Mix the Dry Ingredients:** In a large mixing bowl, whisk together the coconut flour, baking soda, and salt.

3. **Add the Wet Ingredients:** In a separate bowl, whisk together the eggs, melted coconut oil, honey (if using), and apple cider vinegar.

4. **Combine and Form Biscuits:** Add the wet and dry ingredients and stir until a dough forms. The dough will be thick. Scoop out portions of the dough and form into biscuit shapes, placing them on the prepared baking sheet.

5. **Bake:** Bake for 12-15 minutes until the biscuits are golden brown and a toothpick inserted into the center comes clean.

6. **Cool and Serve:** Allow the biscuits to cool slightly on the baking sheet before serving warm.

Chef's Tips

- **Serving Suggestion:** These biscuits are deliciously served with a pat of butter, a drizzle of honey, or alongside eggs and bacon.

- **Storage:** Store any leftovers in an airtight container at room temperature for up to 3 days.

Nutritional Information

Calories: 150 (per biscuit) | Protein: 4g | Total Fat: 12g | Saturated Fat: 9g | Cholesterol: 110mg | Sodium: 150mg | Fiber: 3g

Serving

- **With Toppings:** Serve with butter, honey, or your favorite jam.

- **As a Side,** Pair it with scrambled eggs or breakfast sausage for a complete breakfast.

Chapter 2

Lunch recipes

Mediterranean Chicken Salad with Olive Oil Dressing

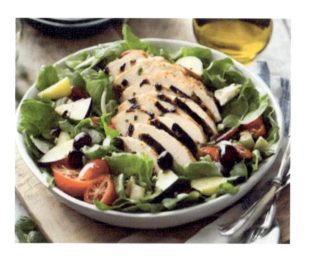

This Mediterranean-inspired chicken salad is a light, refreshing dish perfect for lunch. Packed with fresh vegetables, grilled chicken, and a tangy olive oil dressing, it's a meal that's as nutritious as it is delicious.

Ingredients

- 2 grilled chicken breasts, sliced
- 4 cups mixed greens (such as arugula, spinach, and romaine)
- 1 cup cherry tomatoes, halved
- 1 cucumber, sliced
- 1/2 cup Kalamata olives, pitted and halved
- 1/4 cup feta cheese, crumbled
- 1/4 cup extra virgin olive oil
- 2 tablespoons fresh lemon juice
- 1 teaspoon dried oregano
- Salt and pepper to taste

Instructions

1. **Prepare the Salad Base:** In a large bowl, combine the mixed greens, cherry tomatoes, cucumber, olives, and feta cheese.

2. **Make the Dressing:** In a small bowl, whisk the olive oil, lemon juice, oregano, salt, and pepper until well combined.

3. **Assemble the Salad:** Drizzle the dressing over the salad and toss to coat evenly.

4. **Add the Chicken:** Top the salad with the sliced grilled chicken.

5. **Serve:** Serve immediately as a satisfying, balanced lunch.

Chef's Tips

- **Grilling Tip:** Marinate the chicken breasts in olive oil, lemon juice, garlic, and herbs before grilling for added flavor.

- **Serving Suggestion:** This salad pairs well with whole-grain bread or a small quinoa bowl.

Nutritional Information

Calories: 400 | Protein: 35g | Total Fat: 28g | Saturated Fat: 7g | Cholesterol: 85mg | Sodium: 600mg | Fiber: 4g

Serving:

- **With Bread:** Serve with a slice of whole-grain bread for added fiber and satiety.

- **As a Wrap:** Use the salad as a filling for a whole-grain wrap for a portable lunch option.

Grass-fed beef Burgers with Homemade Ghee

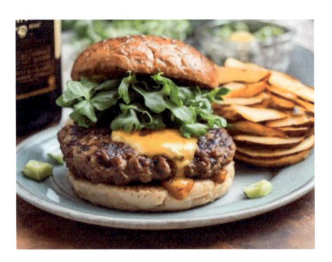

These juicy grass-fed beef burgers are cooked in rich, flavorful ghee, making them a delicious and nutritious lunch option. Whether served on a lettuce wrap or a whole-grain bun, they are sure to satisfy.

Ingredients

- 1 pound grass-fed ground beef

- 2 tablespoons ghee

- Salt and pepper to taste

- 4 lettuce leaves or whole-grain buns

- 1 tomato, sliced

- 1 avocado, sliced

- Optional toppings: cheese, pickles, onions, mustard

Instructions

1. **Form the Patties:** Divide the ground beef into four equal portions and shape them into patties. Season each patty with salt and pepper.

2. **Cook the Burgers:** Heat the ghee in a skillet over medium heat. Add the patties to the skillet and cook for about 4 minutes on each side until they reach your desired level of doneness.

3. **Prepare the Toppings:** While the burgers are cooking, prepare your desired toppings (slice the tomato, avocado, etc.).

4. **Assemble the Burgers:** Serve the patties on lettuce leaves or buns, topped with tomato, avocado, and any additional toppings you prefer.

5. **Serve:** Enjoy immediately with your choice of side.

Chef's Tips

- **Ghee for Cooking:** Ghee has a high smoke point, making it ideal for searing and cooking the burgers to perfection.

- **Topping Variations:** Add your favorite cheese or condiments to customize your burger.

Nutritional Information

Calories: 450 | Protein: 25g | Total Fat: 35g | Saturated Fat: 15g | Cholesterol: 100mg | Sodium: 350mg | Fiber: 4g

Serving:

- **With Fries:** Serve with sweet potato fries or a simple green salad.

- **As a Lettuce Wrap:** For a low-carb option, wrap the burger in lettuce leaves instead of bun.

Wild-caught tuna Salad with Avocado Oil Mayo

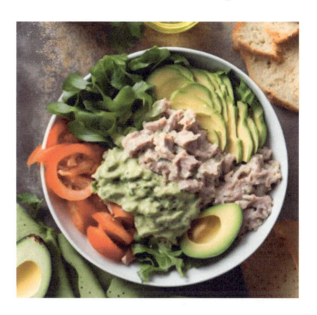

This creamy tuna salad is made with wild-caught tuna and avocado oil mayonnaise, offering a healthier twist on a classic favorite. It's perfect for sandwiches, lettuce wraps, or salad toppings.

Ingredients

- 2 cans of wild-caught tuna, drained

- 1/4 cup avocado oil mayonnaise

- 1 celery stalk, diced

- 1 tablespoon fresh dill, chopped

- 1 tablespoon fresh lemon juice

- Salt and pepper to taste

Instructions

1. **Prepare the Salad:** In a medium bowl, combine the drained tuna, avocado oil mayonnaise, diced celery, chopped dill, and lemon juice.

2. **Season to Taste:** Add salt and pepper to taste, and mix until all ingredients are well combined.

3. **Serve:** Use the tuna salad as a filling for sandwiches or lettuce wraps, or enjoy it alone.

Chef's Tips

- **Mayo Choice:** Avocado oil mayonnaise adds a healthy fat profile and a creamy texture to the tuna salad.

- **Herb Variations:** Substitute dill with parsley or chives for a different flavor profile.

Nutritional Information

Calories: 250 | Protein: 20g | Total Fat: 18g | Saturated Fat: 2g | Cholesterol: 40mg | Sodium: 300mg | Fiber: 1g

Serving:

- **On a Sandwich:** Serve on whole-grain bread with lettuce and tomato.

- **As a Salad Topper:** Use the tuna salad as a topping for a green salad for a light and refreshing lunch.

Roasted Vegetable Quinoa Bowl with Tahini Dressing

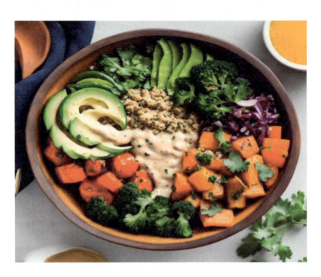

This roasted vegetable quinoa bowl is a hearty and nutritious lunch option. It features a variety of roasted vegetables, protein-packed quinoa, and a creamy tahini dressing. It's a filling meal that's both satisfying and delicious.

Ingredients

- 1 cup quinoa, cooked according to package instructions
- 1 zucchini, sliced
- 1 red bell pepper, chopped
- 1 sweet potato, diced
- 2 tablespoons olive oil
- Salt and pepper to taste
- 1/4 cup tahini
- 2 tablespoons lemon juice
- 1 garlic clove, minced
- Water, as needed for thinning

Instructions

1. **Preheat the Oven:** Preheat your oven to 400°F (200°C).

2. **Roast the Vegetables:** Toss the zucchini, red bell pepper, and sweet potato with

olive oil, salt, and pepper. Spread the vegetables on a baking sheet and roast for 20-25 minutes or until tender and slightly caramelized.

3. **Make the Tahini Dressing:** In a small bowl, whisk together the tahini, lemon juice, minced garlic, and enough water to reach a drizzling consistency.

4. **Assemble the Bowl:** Divide the cooked quinoa into bowls. Top with the roasted vegetables and drizzle with tahini dressing.

5. **Serve:** If desired, serve warm or at room temperature, garnished with fresh parsley or a sprinkle of sesame seeds.

Chef's Tips

- **Veggie Options:** You can swap out the vegetables for whatever you have on hand, such as Brussels sprouts or cauliflower.

- **Tahini Tip:** If your tahini is too thick, warm it slightly or add more lemon juice to make mixing easier.

Nutritional Information

Calories: 450 | Protein: 12g | Total Fat: 20g | Saturated Fat: 3g | Cholesterol: 0mg | Sodium: 300mg | Fiber: 8g

Serving

- **With Greens:** Serve over a bed of spinach or mixed greens for added texture and nutrition.

- **As a Side Dish:** This quinoa bowl also works well as a side dish for grilled meats or fish.

Zucchini Noodles with Pesto and Chicken

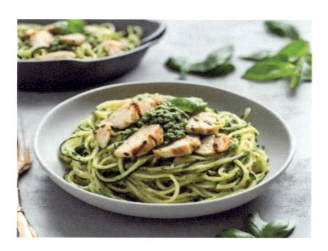

Zucchini noodles, or "zoodles," offer a light and fresh alternative to traditional pasta. Tossed with homemade pesto and grilled chicken, this dish is both low-carb and flavorful.

Ingredients

- 2 medium zucchinis, spiralized into noodles

- 1 grilled chicken breast, sliced

- 1/4 cup homemade or store-bought pesto

- 1 tablespoon olive oil

- Salt and pepper to taste

Instructions

1. **Prepare the Zoodles:** Spiralize the zucchini into noodles using a spiralizer or vegetable peeler.

2. **Cook the Zoodles:** Heat the olive oil in a skillet over medium heat. Add the zucchini noodles and sauté for 2-3 minutes until slightly softened but still al dente.

3. **Add the Pesto:** Toss the zoodles with the pesto until evenly coated—season with salt and pepper to taste.

4. **Top with Chicken:** Place the sliced grilled chicken on the pesto-coated zoodles.

5. **Serve:** Serve immediately as a light and refreshing lunch.

Chef's Tips

- **Pesto Options:** Try using different types of pesto, such as sun-dried tomato or arugula pesto, for a change in flavor.

- **Zoodle Texture:** Avoid overcooking the zucchini noodles to maintain their slightly crunchy texture.

Nutritional Information

Calories: 350 | Protein: 30g | Total Fat: 22g | Saturated Fat: 4g | Cholesterol: 70mg | Sodium: 400mg | Fiber: 4g

Serving

- **With Salad:** Pair with a simple side salad or Caprese salad for a complete meal.

- **As a Pasta Alternative,** Substitute traditional pasta with zucchini noodles in your favorite pasta recipes for a lower-carb option.

Spinach and Goat Cheese Stuffed Chicken Breast

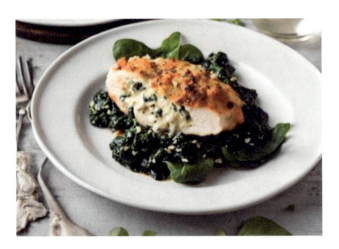

This spinach and goat cheese stuffed chicken breast is a flavorful and elegant dish that's surprisingly easy to prepare. The creamy goat cheese and sautéed spinach make a delicious filling that elevates simple chicken breasts to a gourmet level.

Ingredients

- 4 boneless, skinless chicken breasts

- 4 ounces goat cheese, softened

- 2 cups fresh spinach, chopped

- 1 garlic clove, minced

- 1 tablespoon olive oil

- Salt and pepper to taste

- 1 teaspoon paprika (optional)

Instructions

1. **Preheat the Oven:** Preheat your oven to 375°F (190°C).

2. **Prepare the Filling:** Heat olive oil in a skillet over medium heat. Add the minced garlic and sauté until fragrant. Add the

chopped spinach and cook until wilted. Remove from heat and let cool slightly. Mix the sautéed spinach with the softened goat cheese.

3. **Stuff the Chicken Breasts:** Using a sharp knife carefully cut a pocket into each chicken breast. Stuff each breast with the spinach and goat cheese mixture, then secure with toothpicks if necessary. Season the outside of the chicken breasts with salt, pepper, and paprika if using.

4. **Sear the Chicken:** Heat a little more olive oil over medium-high heat in an oven-safe skillet. Sear the stuffed chicken breasts on each side until golden brown, about 2-3 minutes per side.

5. **Bake:** Transfer the skillet to the preheated oven and bake for 20-25 minutes until the chicken is cooked and reaches an internal temperature of 165°F (75°C).

6. **Serve:** Remove the toothpicks, slice the chicken breasts, and serve warm.

Chef's Tips

- **Securing the Filling:** Use toothpicks to help keep the filling inside the chicken during cooking.

- **Cheese Substitutions:** You can substitute the goat cheese with feta or cream cheese for a different flavor profile.

Nutritional Information:

Calories: 400 | Protein: 40g | Total Fat: 22g | Saturated Fat: 8g | Cholesterol: 120mg | Sodium: 300mg | Fiber: 1g

Serving:

- **With Veggies:** Serve with roasted vegetables or a simple green salad for a balanced meal.

- **Over Pasta:** Slice the chicken and serve over whole-grain pasta with a drizzle of olive oil.

Cobb Salad with Olive Oil and Red Wine Vinaigrette

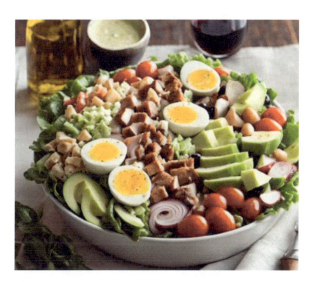

The Cobb salad is a classic American dish known for its hearty mix of ingredients, including grilled chicken, bacon, eggs, and avocado. This version is topped with homemade olive oil and red wine vinaigrette, making it both satisfying and healthy.

Ingredients

- 2 grilled chicken breasts, diced

- 4 slices bacon, cooked and crumbled

- 4 hard-boiled eggs, sliced

- 1 avocado, sliced

- 1 cup cherry tomatoes, halved

- 1/2 cup blue cheese, crumbled

- 4 cups romaine lettuce, chopped

- 1/4 cup extra virgin olive oil

- 2 tablespoons red wine vinegar

- 1 teaspoon Dijon mustard

- Salt and pepper to taste

Instructions

1. **Assemble the Salad:** In a large salad bowl or on a platter, layer the romaine lettuce, grilled chicken, bacon, eggs, avocado, cherry tomatoes, and blue cheese.

2. **Make the Vinaigrette:** In a small bowl, whisk together the olive oil, red wine vinegar, Dijon mustard, salt, and pepper until emulsified.

3. **Dress the Salad:** Drizzle the vinaigrette over the salad just before serving, and toss lightly to combine.

4. **Serve:** Serve immediately as a complete and hearty lunch.

Chef's Tips

- **Meal Prep:** Prepare the ingredients ahead of time and store them separately to assemble the salad quickly during the week.

- **Cheese Substitution:** If you prefer, swap the blue cheese for feta or goat cheese.

Nutritional Information

Calories: 550 | Protein: 35g | Total Fat: 40g | Saturated Fat: 12g | Cholesterol: 300mg | Sodium: 800mg | Fiber: 6g

Serving

- **With Croutons:** Add homemade whole-grain croutons for extra crunch.

- **As a Wrap:** Use the salad as a filling for a whole-grain wrap for a portable lunch option.

Turkey Lettuce Wraps with Avocado Cream

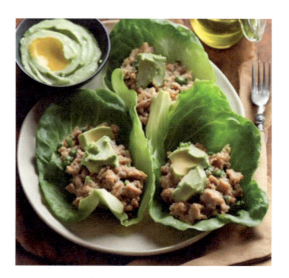

These turkey lettuce wraps are a light, refreshing lunch option, filled with seasoned ground turkey and topped with creamy avocado sauce. They're perfect for a low-carb, high-protein meal that's easy to prepare.

Ingredients

- 1 pound ground turkey

- 1 tablespoon olive oil

- 1 garlic clove, minced

- 1 teaspoon ground cumin

- 1 teaspoon chili powder

- Salt and pepper to taste

- 8 large lettuce leaves (such as romaine or butter lettuce)

- 1 avocado, mashed

- 2 tablespoons Greek yogurt

- 1 tablespoon lime juice

- Fresh cilantro, chopped (for garnish)

Instructions

1. **Cook the Turkey:** Heat olive oil in a skillet over medium heat. Add the minced garlic and sauté until fragrant. Add the ground turkey, cumin, chili powder, salt, and pepper. Cook until the turkey is fully browned and cooked through, about 8-10 minutes.

2. **Prepare the Avocado Cream:** Mash the avocado in a small bowl and mix with Greek yogurt, lime juice, salt, and pepper until smooth.

3. **Assemble the Wraps:** Spoon the cooked turkey mixture onto the center of each lettuce leaf. Top with a dollop of avocado cream and garnish with fresh cilantro.

4. **Serve:** Serve immediately as a light, satisfying lunch.

Chef's Tips

- **Spice Level:** Adjust the spice level by adding more chili powder or a dash of hot sauce.

- **Lettuce Choice:** Use sturdy leaves like romaine or butter lettuce to hold the fillings better.

Nutritional Information

Calories: 300 | Protein: 28g | Total Fat: 18g | Saturated Fat: 4g | Cholesterol: 80mg | Sodium: 400mg | Fiber: 6g

Serving

- **With Salsa:** Serve with a side of salsa or pico de gallo for extra flavor.

- **As a Bowl:** Turn this into a turkey taco bowl by serving the filling over a bed of cauliflower rice or shredded lettuce.

Grilled Shrimp and Avocado Salad

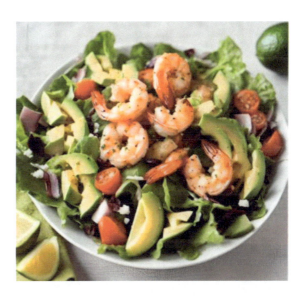

This grilled shrimp and avocado salad is a fresh and vibrant lunch option. It combines the smoky flavor of grilled shrimp with creamy avocado and crisp vegetables. It's light yet satisfying, making it perfect for a midday meal.

Ingredients

- 1 pound large shrimp, peeled and deveined
- 2 tablespoons olive oil

- 1 garlic clove, minced
- 1 teaspoon smoked paprika
- Salt and pepper to taste
- 4 cups mixed greens (such as arugula, spinach, and romaine)
- 1 avocado, sliced
- 1 cup cherry tomatoes, halved
- 1/4 red onion, thinly sliced
- 1/4 cup extra virgin olive oil (for dressing)
- 2 tablespoons fresh lemon juice (for dressing)
- Salt and pepper to taste (for dressing)

Instructions

1. **Marinate the Shrimp:** In a bowl, combine the shrimp with olive oil, minced garlic, smoked paprika, salt, and pepper. Let marinate for 10-15 minutes.

2. **Grill the Shrimp:** Preheat a grill or grill pan over medium heat. Grill the shrimp for 2-3 minutes per side or until opaque and cooked through.

3. **Prepare the Salad:** In a large bowl, combine the mixed greens, avocado slices, cherry tomatoes, and red onion.

4. **Make the Dressing:** In a small bowl, whisk together the olive oil, lemon juice, salt, and pepper.

5. **Assemble the Salad:** Top the salad with the grilled shrimp and drizzle it with lemon vinaigrette.

6. **Serve:** Serve immediately for a fresh and flavorful lunch.

Chef's Tips

- **Grilling Tip:** If you don't have a grill, you can sauté the shrimp in a skillet instead.

- **Dressing Variations:** Add a teaspoon of Dijon mustard or a pinch of red pepper flavor; try for additional flavor.

Nutritional Information

Calories: 350 | Protein: 22g | Saturated Fat: 3g | Cholesterol: 220mg | Sodium: 450mg | Fiber: 7g

Serving

- **With Bread:** Serve with a slice of whole-grain bread or a side of quinoa for added texture.

- **As a Wrap:** Use the salad as a wrap or pita pocket filling.

Cauliflower Rice Stir-Fry with Coconut Aminos

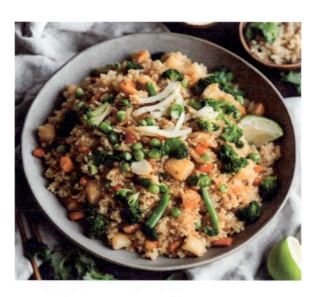

This cauliflower rice stir-fry is a healthy and low-carb alternative to traditional rice dishes, packed with vegetables and seasoned with coconut aminos for a savory, umami flavor. It's a quick and easy lunch that's both nutritious and delicious.

Ingredients

- 4 cups cauliflower rice (store-bought or homemade)
- 1 red bell pepper, diced
- 1 small carrot, julienned
- 1/2 cup snap peas, trimmed
- 2 tablespoons coconut aminos
- 1 tablespoon sesame oil
- 2 garlic cloves, minced
- 1-inch piece of ginger, minced
- 2 eggs, lightly beaten
- Salt and pepper to taste
- Sliced green onions and sesame seeds for garnish

Instructions

1. **Prepare the Vegetables:** Heat the sesame oil in a large skillet or wok over medium heat. Add the minced garlic and ginger, and sauté until fragrant.

2. **Cook the Vegetables:** Add the red bell pepper, carrot, and snap peas to the skillet. Cook for 3-4 minutes until the vegetables are slightly tender.

3. **Add the Cauliflower Rice:** Stir in the cauliflower rice and cook for another 3-4 minutes until the rice is heated.

4. **Scramble the Eggs:** Push the cauliflower rice mixture to one side of the skillet. Pour the beaten eggs into the empty side and scramble until cooked. Mix the eggs into the rice.

5. **Season and Serve:** Stir in the coconut aminos and season with salt and pepper to taste. Garnish with sliced green onions and sesame seeds.

Chef's Tips

- **Protein Addition:** Add cooked chicken, shrimp, or tofu for extra protein.

- **Vegetable Variations:** Feel free to swap out or add any vegetables you like, such as broccoli or mushrooms.

Nutritional Information

Calories: 200 | Protein: 10g | Total Fat: 12g | Saturated Fat: 2g | Cholesterol: 140mg | Sodium: 400mg | Fiber: 5g

Serving:

- **With Protein:** Serve alongside grilled chicken or tofu for a more substantial meal.

- **As a Side Dish,** Pair with your favorite Asian-inspired main dish for a complete meal.

Chicken Caesar Salad with Homemade Dressing

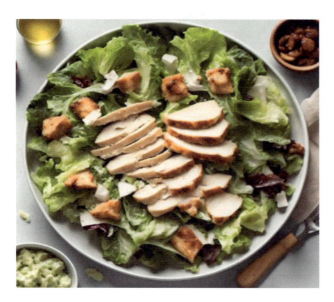

This chicken Caesar salad features tender grilled chicken, crisp romaine lettuce, and a rich, creamy homemade Caesar dressing. It's a classic lunch option that's satisfying and easy to prepare.

Ingredients

- 2 grilled chicken breasts, sliced
- 4 cups romaine lettuce, chopped
- 1/4 cup grated Parmesan cheese
- 1/4 cup croutons (optional)
- 1/4 cup extra virgin olive oil (for dressing)
- 1 egg yolk
- 2 anchovy fillets, minced
- 1 garlic clove, minced
- 1 teaspoon Dijon mustard
- 1 tablespoon lemon juice
- Salt and pepper to taste

Instructions

1. **Prepare the Dressing:** In a bowl, whisk together the egg yolk, minced anchovy fillets, garlic, Dijon mustard, lemon juice, and olive oil until emulsified—season with salt and pepper to taste.

2. **Assemble the Salad:** In a large salad bowl, toss the chopped romaine lettuce with the Parmesan cheese, croutons (if using), and sliced grilled chicken.

3. **Dress the Salad:** Drizzle the homemade Caesar dressing over the salad and toss to coat evenly.

4. **Serve:** Serve immediately as a hearty, flavorful lunch.

Chef's Tips

- **Dressing Variations:** If you prefer a lighter dressing, add a little water to thin it out.

- **Anchovy Substitute:** If you don't like anchovies, you can omit them, though they add a traditional Caesar flavor.

Nutritional Information

Calories: 450 | Protein: 35g | Total Fat: 30g | Saturated Fat: 7g | Cholesterol: 200mg | Sodium: 600mg | Fiber: 3g

Serving

- **With Bread:** Serve with a slice of garlic bread or whole-grain toast.

- **As a Wrap:** Use the salad as a filling for a Caesar salad wrap with a whole-grain tortilla.

Baked Cod with Lemon Butter Sauce

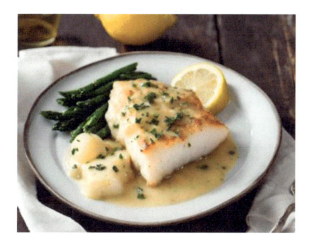

This baked cod with lemon butter sauce is a light and flavorful dish that's quick to prepare. The tender cod fillets are baked to perfection and topped with a simple yet delicious lemon butter sauce, making it a perfect lunch option.

Ingredients

- 4 cod fillets
- 4 tablespoons butter (preferably grass-fed)
- 2 garlic cloves, minced
- Juice of 1 lemon
- Zest of 1 lemon
- 1 tablespoon fresh parsley, chopped
- Salt and pepper to taste
- Lemon wedges for serving

Instructions

1. **Preheat the Oven:** Preheat your oven to 400°F (200°C). Line a baking sheet with parchment paper.

2. **Prepare the Cod:** Pat the cod fillets dry with paper towels. Place them on the prepared baking sheet and season with salt and pepper.

3. **Bake the Cod:** Bake the cod fillets for 12-15 minutes or until the fish is opaque and flakes easily with a fork.

4. **Make the Lemon Butter Sauce:** While the cod is baking, melt the butter in a small saucepan over medium heat. Add the minced garlic and sauté until fragrant. Stir in the lemon juice and zest, and cook for 1-2 minutes. Remove from heat and stir in the chopped parsley.

5. **Serve:** Drizzle the lemon butter sauce over the baked cod fillets and serve immediately with lemon wedges on the side.

Chef's Tips

- **Butter Sauce Variations:** Add a splash of white wine or a pinch of red pepper flakes to the lemon butter sauce for a more intense flavor.

- **Cod Substitutions:** This recipe works well with other white fish like halibut or haddock.

Nutritional Information

Calories: 300 | Protein: 25g | Total Fat: 20g | Saturated Fat: 12g | Cholesterol: 90mg | Sodium: 400mg | Fiber: 0g

Serving

- **With Vegetables:** Serve with steamed asparagus or roasted Brussels sprouts for a complete meal.

- **With Rice:** Pair with cauliflower or quinoa for added texture and nutrition.

Eggplant Parmesan with Almond Flour

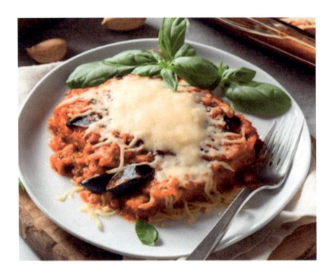

This eggplant Parmesan is a healthier, gluten-free version of the classic Italian dish. Made with almond flour instead of breadcrumbs, it's crispy, flavorful, and perfect for a satisfying lunch.

Ingredients

- 2 large eggplants, sliced into 1/4-inch rounds
- 2 cups almond flour
- 2 eggs, beaten
- 1 cup marinara sauce
- 1 cup mozzarella cheese, shredded
- 1/2 cup Parmesan cheese, grated
- 1 tablespoon dried oregano
- 1 tablespoon olive oil
- Salt and pepper to taste
- Fresh basil for garnish

Instructions

1. **Preheat the Oven:** Preheat your oven to 375°F (190°C). Line a baking sheet with parchment paper and lightly grease it with olive oil.

2. **Prepare the Eggplant:** Sprinkle the eggplant slices with salt and let them sit for 15 minutes to draw out excess moisture. Pat them dry with paper towels.

3. **Bread the Eggplant:** Set up a breading station with almond flour in one bowl and beaten eggs in another. Dip each eggplant slice into the egg, then coat with almond flour.

4. **Bake the Eggplant:** Arrange the breaded slices on the prepared baking sheet. Bake for 20 minutes, flipping halfway through, until the eggplant is golden and crispy.

5. **Assemble the Dish:** In a baking dish, layer the baked eggplant slices with marinara sauce, mozzarella, and Parmesan cheese. Repeat the layers, ending with cheese on top. Sprinkle with dried oregano.

6. **Bake:** Bake the assembled dish for 20-25 minutes or until the cheese is melted and bubbly.

7. **Serve:** Garnish with fresh basil and serve warm.

Chef's Tips

- **Marinara Sauce:** Use a high-quality, low-sugar marinara sauce for the best flavor.

- **Cheese Options:** Add ricotta cheese between the layers for a richer flavor.

Nutritional Information

Serving:

- **With Salad:** Serve alongside a fresh green salad with balsamic vinaigrette.

- **As a Side,** Pair it with grilled chicken or fish for a more substantial meal.

Pulled Pork Lettuce Wraps with Salsa Verde

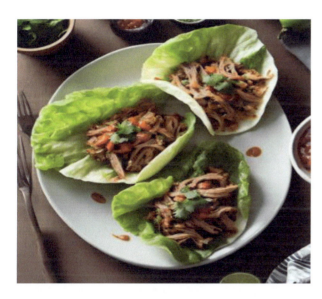

These pulled pork lettuce wraps are a flavorful, low-carb lunch option that's both light and satisfying. Topped with a zesty salsa verde, they're perfect for those looking to enjoy a hearty meal without the heaviness of bread or tortillas.

Ingredients

- 1 pound cooked pulled pork (leftovers or store-bought)

- 8 large lettuce leaves (such as romaine or butter lettuce)

- 1 cup salsa verde (homemade or store-bought)

- 1 avocado, sliced

- 1/4 cup red onion, thinly sliced

- Fresh cilantro, chopped (for garnish)

- Lime wedges for serving

Instructions

1. **Reheat the Pulled Pork:** Reheat leftover pulled pork in a skillet over medium heat until warmed.

2. **Assemble the Wraps:** Lay the lettuce leaves flat and fill each with a portion of pulled pork. Top with salsa verde, avocado slices, and red onion.

3. **Garnish and Serve:** Garnish with fresh cilantro and serve with lime wedges on the side.

Chef's Tips

- **Pork Preparation:** If making your own pulled pork, consider slow-cooking a pork shoulder with spices like cumin, paprika, and garlic.

- **Lettuce Choice:** Use sturdy leaves to hold the fillings better without tearing.

Nutritional Information

Serving

- **With Sides:** Serve with a side of cauliflower rice or a simple tomato salad.

- **As Tacos:** Use small corn tortillas instead of lettuce wraps for a different presentation.

Greek Salad with Feta and Kalamata Olives

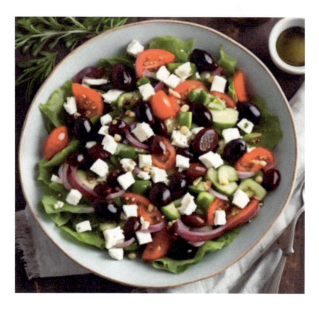

This classic Greek salad is a vibrant and refreshing dish featuring crisp vegetables, briny Kalamata olives, and creamy feta cheese. It's a light yet flavorful lunch, perfect for a warm day.

Ingredients

- 4 cups romaine lettuce, chopped
- 1 cucumber, sliced
- 1 cup cherry tomatoes, halved
- 1/2 red onion, thinly sliced
- 1/2 cup Kalamata olives, pitted and halved
- 1/2 cup feta cheese, crumbled
- 1/4 cup extra virgin olive oil
- 2 tablespoons red wine vinegar
- 1 teaspoon dried oregano
- Salt and pepper to taste

Instructions

1. **Prepare the Salad:** In a large bowl, combine the chopped romaine lettuce, cucumber slices, cherry tomatoes, red onion, and Kalamata olives.

2. **Make the Dressing:** In a small bowl, whisk together the olive oil, red wine vinegar, oregano, salt, and pepper until well combined.

3. **Toss the Salad:** Drizzle the dressing over the salad and toss to coat evenly.

4. **Add the Feta:** Sprinkle the crumbled feta cheese over the top of the salad.

5. **Serve:** Serve immediately as a fresh and flavorful lunch.

Chef's Tips

- **Olive Variety:** Add a mix of different olives, such as green or black, for a more complex flavor.

- **Dressing Tip:** Whisk in a tablespoon of Greek yogurt for a creamier dressing.

Nutritional Information

Calories: 300 | Protein: 8g | Total Fat: 25g | Saturated Fat: 8g | Cholesterol: 25mg | Sodium: 700mg | Fiber: 4g

Serving

- **With Pita:** Serve with warm pita bread or chips for added texture.

- **As a Side,** Pair it with grilled chicken or lamb for a complete Mediterranean-inspired meal.

Chapter 3

Dinner

The Importance of a Satisfying Evening Meal

Dinner is more than just the last meal of the day; it's an opportunity to nourish your body and bring closure to your day with a satisfying and balanced meal. A well-planned dinner can help stabilize blood sugar levels overnight, support restful sleep, and energize you. In this chapter, we focus on dinner recipes that are both delicious and designed to provide the nutrients your body needs to repair and rejuvenate while you rest.

A satisfying evening meal should include a good balance of protein, healthy fats, and fiber-rich vegetables. These components work together to keep you full, support digestion, and promote overall health. Whether you're preparing a quick weeknight dinner or a more elaborate meal for the weekend, these recipes are crafted to be both enjoyable and nutritious.

Cooking with Fats that Support Health

In this chapter, you'll find recipes that make the most of healthy, traditional fats like butter, olive oil, ghee, and coconut oil. These fats add flavor and richness to your meals and provide essential nutrients that support heart health, brain function, and overall well-being. By choosing the right fats, you can create satisfying and health-promoting dinners.

Garlic Butter Steak with Roasted Vegetables

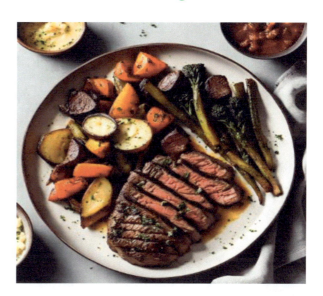

This garlic butter steak is a perfect dinner option for those who enjoy a rich, flavorful meal. Paired with a medley of roasted vegetables, it offers a balanced and satisfying evening meal that's both delicious and nutritious.

Ingredients

- 2 ribeye or sirloin steaks
- 4 tablespoons butter (preferably grass-fed)
- 4 garlic cloves, minced
- 1 teaspoon fresh thyme leaves
- 1 bunch asparagus, trimmed
- 1 red bell pepper, sliced
- 1 zucchini, sliced
- 2 tablespoons olive oil
- Salt and pepper to taste
- Fresh parsley, chopped (for garnish)

Instructions

1. **Prepare the Vegetables:** Preheat your oven to 400°F (200°C). Toss the asparagus, bell pepper, and zucchini with olive oil, salt, and pepper. Spread them on a baking sheet and roast for 20-25 minutes until tender and slightly caramelized.

2. **Cook the Steaks:** Season the steaks with salt and pepper. Heat a large skillet over medium-high heat and add the steaks. Cook for 4-5 minutes on each side until they reach your desired level. Remove from the skillet and let them rest.

3. **Make the Garlic Butter:** Melt the butter in the same skillet over medium heat. Add the minced garlic and thyme, cooking until the garlic is fragrant and slightly golden.

4. **Serve:** Pour the garlic butter over the steaks and serve alongside the roasted vegetables. Garnish with fresh parsley.

Chef's Tips

- **Steak Resting:** Letting the steak rest after cooking allows the juices to redistribute, ensuring a juicy and flavorful result.

- **Vegetable Options:** You can swap in your favorite vegetables, such as carrots, Brussels sprouts, or mushrooms.

Nutritional Information

Calories: 650 | Protein: 45g | Total Fat: 50g | Saturated Fat: 20g | Cholesterol: 160mg | Sodium: 450mg | Fiber: 6g

Serving

- **With Potatoes:** Serve with roasted potatoes or mashed cauliflower for a more substantial meal.

- **As a Salad,** Slice the steak and serve over a bed of arugula or mixed greens for a lighter option.

Baked Salmon with Lemon Herb Ghee Sauce

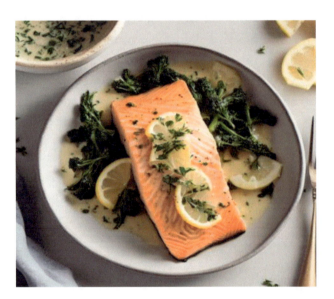

This baked salmon dish is simple yet elegant. It features a tangy lemon herb ghee sauce that enhances the salmon's natural flavor. It's an easy-to-make dinner that's both healthy and full of flavor.

Ingredients

- 4 salmon fillets

- 4 tablespoons ghee

- Juice and zest of 1 lemon

- 2 garlic cloves, minced

- 1 tablespoon fresh dill, chopped

- 1 tablespoon fresh parsley, chopped

- Salt and pepper to taste

- Lemon wedges for serving

Instructions

1. **Preheat the Oven:** Preheat your oven to 375°F (190°C). Line a baking sheet with parchment paper.

2. **Prepare the Salmon:** Place the salmon fillets on the prepared baking sheet—season with salt and pepper.

3. **Make the Lemon Herb Ghee Sauce:** Melt the ghee in a small saucepan over medium heat. Add the garlic and cook until fragrant. Stir in the lemon juice, zest, dill, and parsley.

4. **Bake the Salmon:** Pour the lemon herb ghee sauce over the salmon fillets. Bake for 15-20 minutes until the salmon is cooked and flakes easily with a fork.

5. **Serve:** Serve the salmon with additional lemon wedges and garnish with fresh herbs.

Chef's Tips

- **Ghee Alternative:** If you don't have ghee, substitute it with butter or olive oil, though ghee adds a rich, nutty flavor.

- **Salmon Cooking:** To ensure even cooking, bring the salmon to room temperature before baking.

Nutritional Information:

Calories: 400 | Protein: 34g | Total Fat: 28g | Saturated Fat: 12g | Cholesterol: 95mg | Sodium: 350mg | Fiber: 0g

Serving

- **With Vegetables:** Pair with steamed green beans or roasted Brussels sprouts.

- **With Rice:** Serve over cauliflower rice or a side of quinoa for added texture and nutrition.

Chicken Thighs in Coconut Milk Curry

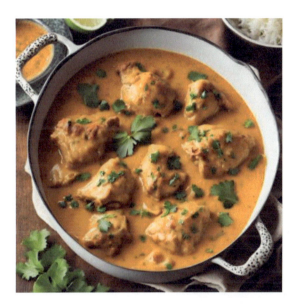

This dish features tender chicken thighs simmered in a creamy coconut milk curry sauce infused with aromatic spices. It's a comforting and flavorful dinner perfect for a cozy night in.

Ingredients

- 6 chicken thighs, bone-in and skin-on

- 1 tablespoon coconut oil

- 1 onion, diced

- 3 garlic cloves, minced

- 1 tablespoon ginger, minced

- 1 tablespoon curry powder

- 1 teaspoon ground turmeric

- 1/2 teaspoon ground cumin

- 1 can (14 ounces) coconut milk

- 1 cup chicken broth

- 1 cup diced tomatoes

- Salt and pepper to taste

- Fresh cilantro for garnish

Instructions

1. **Sear the Chicken:** Heat the coconut oil in a large skillet over medium-high heat. Season the chicken thighs with salt and pepper, and sear them skin-side down until golden brown. Flip and sear the other side. Remove the chicken from the skillet and set aside.

2. **Cook the Aromatics:** In the same skillet, add the diced onion, garlic, and ginger. Sauté until the onion is soft and translucent.

3. **Add the Spices:** Stir in the curry powder, turmeric, and cumin, cooking for 1-2 minutes until the spices are fragrant.

4. **Simmer the Curry:** Add the coconut milk, chicken broth, and diced tomatoes to the skillet. Stir to combine, then return the chicken thighs to the skillet, skin-side up. Bring to a simmer, reduce heat to low, and cover. Cook for 25-30 minutes until the chicken is cooked through.

5. **Serve:** Serve the chicken curry with a sprinkle of fresh cilantro.

Chef's Tips

- **Spice Adjustments:** Adjust the level of curry powder to your taste, adding more or less depending on your spice preference.

- **Thickening the Sauce:** If the sauce is too thin, let it simmer uncovered for a few minutes to reduce and thicken.

Nutritional Information

Calories: 550 | Protein: 35g | Total Fat: 40g | Saturated Fat: 25g | Cholesterol: 120mg | Sodium: 450mg | Fiber: 3g

Serving

- **With Rice:** Serve over steamed jasmine rice or cauliflower rice.

- **With Naan:** Pair with warm naan bread to soak up the delicious curry sauce.

Zucchini Noodles with Pesto and Parmesan

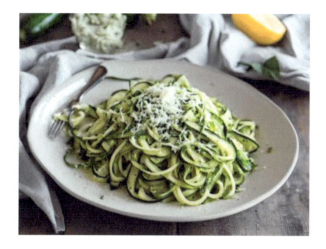

Zucchini noodles, or "zoodles," are a low-carb, nutrient-rich alternative to traditional pasta. Tossed with a vibrant pesto sauce and topped with Parmesan, this dish is light yet satisfying, making it an ideal dinner choice.

Ingredients

- 4 medium zucchinis, spiralized into noodles
- 1/4 cup homemade or store-bought pesto
- 1/4 cup grated Parmesan cheese
- 2 tablespoons olive oil
- 1 garlic clove, minced
- Salt and pepper to taste
- Fresh basil leaves for garnish

Instructions:

1. **Prepare the Zoodles:** Heat olive oil in a large skillet over medium heat. Add the minced garlic and sauté until fragrant.

2. **Cook the Zoodles:** Add the zucchini noodles to the skillet and sauté for 2-3 minutes until slightly softened but still al dente.

3. **Add the Pesto:** Remove the skillet from heat and toss the zoodles with the pesto until evenly coated season with salt and pepper.

4. **Serve:** Divide the zoodles between plates, top with grated Parmesan, and garnish with fresh basil leaves.

Chef's Tips

- **Zoodle Cooking:** Avoid overcooking the zucchini noodles to maintain their texture and prevent them from becoming mushy.

- **Pesto Variations:** Try different types of pesto, such as sun-dried tomato or arugula pesto, for a change in flavor.

Nutritional Information

Calories: 250 | Protein: 8g | Total Fat: 20g | Saturated Fat: 5g | Cholesterol: 15mg | Sodium: 350mg | Fiber: 4g

Serving:

- **With Chicken:** Serve alongside grilled chicken or shrimp for added protein.

- **As a Side Dish,** Pair it with a light salad or roasted vegetables for a complete meal.

Lamb Chops with Mint Yogurt Sauce

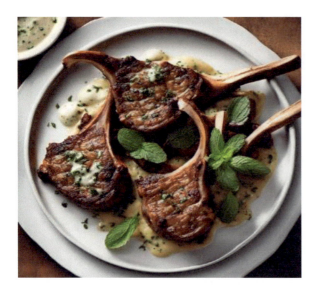

These succulent lamb chops are perfectly seared and served with a refreshing mint yogurt sauce. This dish is a delightful combination of rich flavors and cool, creamy accents, making it an excellent choice for a satisfying dinner.

Ingredients

- 8 lamb chops
- 2 tablespoons olive oil
- 2 garlic cloves, minced
- Salt and pepper to taste
- 1 cup plain Greek yogurt
- 2 tablespoons fresh mint, chopped
- 1 tablespoon lemon juice
- 1 teaspoon honey (optional)

Instructions

1. **Prepare the Lamb Chops:** Season the lamb chops with salt, pepper, and minced garlic. Heat the olive oil in a large skillet over medium-high heat. Add the lamb chops and sear for 3-4 minutes per side until they reach your desired doneness.

2. **Make the Mint Yogurt Sauce:** In a small bowl, combine the Greek yogurt, chopped mint, lemon juice, and honey. Mix until smooth and well combined.

3. **Serve:** Serve the lamb chops hot, with the mint yogurt sauce on the side or drizzled over the top.

Chef's Tips

- **Lamb Cooking:** For the best results, cook the lamb chops to medium-rare to medium, as overcooking can make them challenging.

- **Mint Yogurt:** The mint yogurt sauce can be prepared and stored in the refrigerator for up to 2 days.

Nutritional Information

Calories: 450 | Protein: 30g | Total Fat: 35g | Saturated Fat: 15g | Cholesterol: 110mg | Sodium: 300mg | Fiber: 0g

Serving

- **With Couscous:** Serve with couscous or quinoa for a Mediterranean-inspired meal.

- **With Vegetables:** Pair with roasted or grilled vegetables, such as asparagus or bell peppers.

Pork Tenderloin with Mustard Cream Sauce

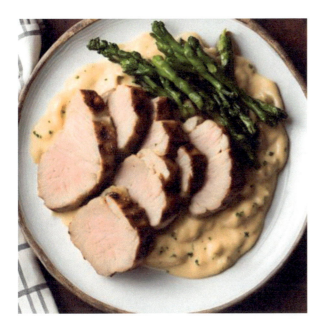

This pork tenderloin dish features succulent, seared tenderloin with rich mustard cream sauce. The tangy, creamy sauce pairs perfectly with the tender pork, making it a delightful option for a satisfying dinner.

Ingredients

- 1 pork tenderloin (about 1 pound)
- 2 tablespoons olive oil
- Salt and pepper to taste
- 1/2 cup heavy cream
- 2 tablespoons Dijon mustard
- 1 teaspoon whole-grain mustard
- 1 garlic clove, minced
- 1 tablespoon fresh thyme leaves
- Fresh parsley, chopped (for garnish)

Instructions

1. **Prepare the Pork Tenderloin:** Preheat your oven to 375°F (190°C). Season the pork tenderloin with salt and pepper.

2. **Sear the Pork:** Heat the olive oil in an oven-safe skillet over medium-high heat. Sear the pork on all sides until golden brown, about 2-3 minutes per side.

3. **Roast the Pork:** Transfer the skillet to the preheated oven and roast the pork for 15-20 minutes, or until the internal temperature reaches 145°F (63°C). Remove the pork from the skillet and let it rest.

4. **Make the Mustard Cream Sauce:** Add minced garlic and sauté until fragrant in the same skillet. Stir in the heavy cream, Dijon mustard, whole grain mustard, and fresh thyme. Simmer for 2-3 minutes until the sauce thickens slightly.

5. **Serve:** Slice the pork tenderloin and serve it with the mustard cream sauce drizzled over the top. Garnish with fresh parsley.

Chef's Tips

- **Resting the Pork:** Letting the pork rest after roasting allows the juices to redistribute, resulting in a more tender and flavorful dish.

- **Sauce Variations:** Add a splash of white wine to the sauce for extra depth of flavor.

Nutritional Information

Calories: 400 | Protein: 30g | Total Fat: 28g | Saturated Fat: 14g | Cholesterol: 120mg | Sodium: 350mg | Fiber: 0g

Serving

- **With Vegetables:** Serve with roasted Brussels sprouts or sautéed green beans.

- **With Potatoes:** Pair with mashed potatoes or roasted sweet potatoes for a complete meal.

Shrimp Scampi with Zoodles

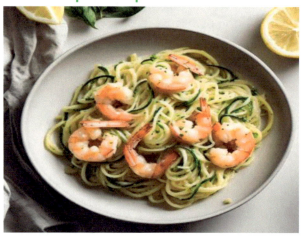

This shrimp scampi dish is a light, flavorful option that substitutes traditional pasta with zucchini noodles (zoodles). The garlic butter sauce complements the tender shrimp and zoodles, making it a delicious and low-carb dinner choice.

Ingredients

- 1 pound large shrimp, peeled and deveined

- 4 medium zucchinis, spiraled into noodles

- 4 tablespoons butter

- 4 garlic cloves, minced

- 1/4 cup white wine (optional)

- Juice of 1 lemon

- 1/4 teaspoon red pepper flakes (optional)

- Salt and pepper to taste

- Fresh parsley, chopped (for garnish)

Instructions

1. **Cook the Shrimp:** Melt 2 tablespoons of butter in a large skillet over medium heat. Add the shrimp and cook on each side for 2-3 minutes until they are pink and opaque. Remove the shrimp from the skillet and set aside.

2. **Make the Scampi Sauce:** Add the remaining butter and minced garlic in the same skillet. Cook until the garlic is fragrant. Add the white wine and let it simmer for 2-3 minutes until slightly reduced. Stir in the lemon juice and red pepper flakes.

3. **Cook the Zoodles:** Add the zucchini noodles to the skillet and toss them in the garlic butter sauce. Cook for 2-3 minutes until the zoodles are tender but still al dente.

4. **Combine and Serve:** Return the cooked shrimp to the skillet and toss to combine season with salt and pepper. Serve immediately, garnished with fresh parsley.

Chef's Tips

- **Zoodle Texture:** To prevent the zoodles from becoming too watery, lightly salt them, sit for a few minutes before cooking, and pat dry.

- **Wine Substitute:** If you prefer not to use wine, substitute with chicken broth or extra lemon juice for added flavor.

Nutritional Information

Calories: 350 | Protein: 30g | Total Fat: 20g | Saturated Fat: 10g | Cholesterol: 240mg | Sodium: 600mg | Fiber: 3g

Serving

- **With Salad:** Pair with a simple Caesar salad or a Caprese salad.

- **As a Side:** Serve with garlic bread or a small portion of cauliflower rice for added texture.

Herb-crusted roast Beef with Garlic Butter

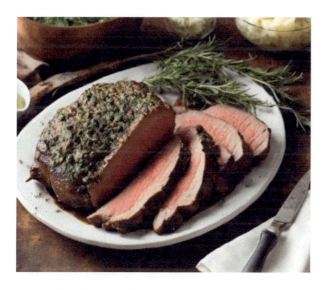

This herb-crusted roast beef is a show-stopping main course, perfect for a special dinner. The meat is coated in a flavorful herb mixture and roasted to perfection, then topped with a rich garlic butter sauce for added indulgence.

Ingredients

- 1 (3-pound) beef roast (such as rib eye or top sirloin)

- 2 tablespoons olive oil

- 4 garlic cloves, minced

- 1 tablespoon fresh rosemary, chopped

- 1 tablespoon fresh thyme, chopped

- 1 tablespoon Dijon mustard

- Salt and pepper to taste

- 4 tablespoons butter, melted

Instructions

1. **Prepare the Beef Roast:** Preheat your oven to 425°F (220°C). Pat the beef roast dry with paper towels. Rub the roast with olive oil, then coat it with the minced garlic, rosemary, thyme, Dijon mustard, salt, and pepper.

2. **Roast the Beef:** Place the roast on a rack in a roasting pan. Roast for 15 minutes at 425°F (220°C), then reduce the heat to 350°F (175°C) and continue roasting for 1-1.5 hours or until the internal temperature reaches your desired level of doneness (130°F for medium-rare).

3. **Make the Garlic Butter:** While the beef is roasting, melt the butter in a small saucepan over medium heat. Stir in any remaining minced garlic and cook until fragrant.

4. **Serve:** Remove the roast from the oven and let it rest for 15-20 minutes before slicing. Serve with the melted garlic butter drizzled over the top.

Chef's Tips

- **Doneness Check:** Use a meat thermometer to check the roast's internal temperature for perfect doneness.

- **Resting the Meat:** Letting the roast rest redistributes the juices, resulting in a more tender and juicy roast.

Nutritional Information

Calories: 600 | Protein: 50g | Total Fat: 45g | Saturated Fat: 20g | Cholesterol: 160mg | Sodium: 500mg | Fiber: 0g

Serving

- **With Potatoes:** Serve with roasted potatoes or mashed cauliflower.

- **With Vegetables:** Pair with roasted carrots, Brussels sprouts, or green beans.

Chicken Marsala with Mushroom Sauce

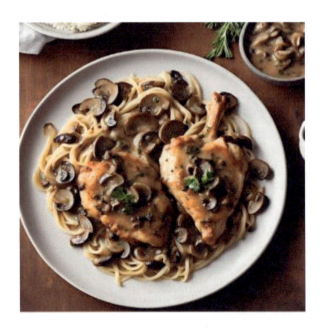

Chicken Marsala is a classic Italian-American dish featuring tender chicken breasts cooked in rich Marsala wine and mushroom sauce. It's a comforting and flavorful dinner option that's easy enough for a weeknight meal but elegant enough for entertaining.

Ingredients

- 4 boneless, skinless chicken breasts

- 1/2 cup all-purpose flour (or almond flour for gluten-free)

- 2 tablespoons olive oil

- 2 tablespoons butter

- 8 ounces mushrooms, sliced

- 2 garlic cloves, minced

- 1/2 cup Marsala wine

- 1/2 cup chicken broth

- 1/4 cup heavy cream (optional)

- Salt and pepper to taste

- Fresh parsley, chopped (for garnish)

Instructions

1. **Prepare the Chicken:** Season the chicken breasts with salt and pepper, then dredge them in flour, shaking off any excess.

2. **Cook the Chicken:** Heat the olive oil in a large skillet over medium heat. Add the chicken breasts and cook for 5-7 minutes per side until golden brown and cooked through. Remove the chicken from the skillet and set aside.

3. **Make the Mushroom Sauce:** Melt the butter in the same skillet and add the sliced mushrooms. Sauté until the mushrooms are browned. Add the minced garlic and cook for another minute.

4. **Add the Marsala and Broth:** Pour in the Marsala wine and chicken broth, scraping up any browned bits from the bottom of the skillet. Simmer for 5 minutes until the

sauce reduces slightly. Stir in the heavy cream for a creamier sauce.

5. **Combine and Serve:** Return the chicken to the skillet, spooning the sauce over the top. Cook for another 2-3 minutes to warm through. Serve garnished with fresh parsley.

Chef's Tips

- **Marsala Wine:** Use dry Marsala wine for a less sweet sauce or sweet Marsala if you prefer a richer flavor.

- **Gluten-Free Option:** Use almond flour instead of all-purpose flour to make the dish gluten-free.

Nutritional Information

Calories: 450 | Protein: 35g | Total Fat: 25g | Saturated Fat: 10g | Cholesterol: 120mg | Sodium: 400mg | Fiber: 2g

Serving:

- **With Pasta:** Serve over whole-grain pasta or zucchini noodles.

- **With Vegetables:** Pair with steamed broccoli or roasted asparagus.

Braised Short Ribs with Red Wine and Vegetables

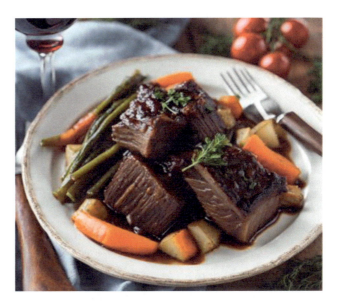

These braised short ribs are cooked slowly in a rich red wine sauce with vegetables until they are tender and fall off the bone. This hearty dish is perfect for a comforting dinner on a fantastic evening, offering deep flavors and a satisfying meal.

Ingredients

- 4 pounds of bone-in beef short ribs
- 2 tablespoons olive oil
- Salt and pepper to taste
- 1 onion, diced
- 3 carrots, peeled and chopped
- 2 celery stalks, chopped
- 4 garlic cloves, minced
- 2 tablespoons tomato paste
- 2 cups red wine
- 2 cups beef broth
- 2 sprigs fresh thyme
- 2 sprigs fresh rosemary
- 2 bay leaves

Instructions

1. **Sear the Short Ribs:** Preheat your oven to 325°F (160°C). Season the short ribs with salt and pepper. Heat olive oil in a large Dutch oven over medium-high heat. Sear the short ribs on all sides until browned, about 8-10 minutes total. Remove and set aside.

2. **Cook the Vegetables:** In the same pot, add the diced onion, carrots, celery, and garlic. Sauté until softened, about 5 minutes. Stir in the tomato paste and cook for another 2 minutes.

3. **Deglaze with Wine:** Pour in the red wine, scraping up any browned bits from the bottom of the pot. Simmer for 5 minutes until the wine reduces slightly.

4. **Add the Broth and Herbs.** Return the short ribs and any accumulated juices to the pot. Add the beef broth, thyme, rosemary, and bay leaves. Bring to a simmer.

5. **Braise in the Oven:** Cover the pot with a lid and transfer to the preheated oven. Braise for 2.5 to 3 hours, or until the short ribs are tender and the meat quickly pulls away from the bone.

6. **Serve:** Remove the short ribs from the pot and discard the herb sprigs and bay leaves. Serve the short ribs with the braising liquid and spoon vegetables over the top.

Chef's Tips

- **Wine Choice:** Use a dry red wine like Cabernet Sauvignon or Merlot for the best flavor in the sauce.

- **Cooking Tip:** The longer the short ribs cook, the more tender they will become, so don't rush the braising process.

Nutritional Information

Calories: 600 | Protein: 40g | Total Fat: 40g | Saturated Fat: 15g | Cholesterol: 150mg | Sodium: 500mg | Fiber: 4g

Serving:

- **With Mashed Potatoes:** Serve over creamy mashed potatoes or polenta to soak up the rich sauce.

- **With Greens:** Pair with sautéed spinach or roasted Brussels sprouts for a balanced meal.

Thai Green Curry with Coconut Milk

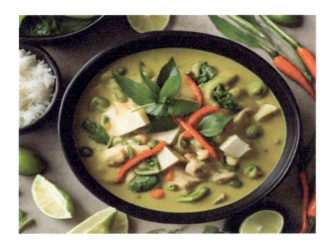

Thai green curry is a fragrant and flavorful dish made with aromatic herbs, spices, and coconut milk. This version includes tender chicken and fresh vegetables, making it a satisfying and nourishing dinner.

Ingredients

- 1 pound chicken thighs or breasts, cut into bite-sized pieces
- 2 tablespoons green curry paste
- 1 can (14 ounces) coconut milk
- 1 tablespoon coconut oil
- 1 onion, sliced
- 2 garlic cloves, minced
- 1-inch piece of ginger, minced
- 1 red bell pepper, sliced
- 1 zucchini, sliced
- 1 cup broccoli florets
- 1 tablespoon fish sauce
- 1 tablespoon lime juice
- Fresh basil leaves for garnish

Instructions

1. **Cook the Aromatics:** Heat the coconut oil in a large skillet or wok over medium heat. Add the sliced onion, garlic, and ginger, and sauté until fragrant and the onion is soft.

2. **Add the Curry Paste:** Stir in the green curry paste and cook for 1-2 minutes until it begins to release its aroma.

3. **Cook the Chicken:** Add the chicken pieces to the skillet until lightly browned on all sides.

4. **Add the Vegetables:** Stir in the coconut milk, fish sauce, and lime juice. Bring to a simmer, then add the bell pepper, zucchini, and broccoli. Cook for 10-15 minutes until the vegetables are tender and the chicken is cooked.

5. **Serve:** Serve the curry hot, garnished with fresh basil leaves.

Chef's Tips

- **Spice Level:** Adjust the amount of curry paste based on your spice tolerance. Start with less and add more as needed.

- **Protein Options:** This curry works well with shrimp, tofu, or beef instead of chicken.

Nutritional Information

Calories: 400 | Protein: 25g | Total Fat: 30g | Saturated Fat: 20g | Cholesterol: 80mg | Sodium: 500mg | Fiber: 4g

Serving

- **With Rice:** Serve over jasmine or cauliflower rice to soak up the delicious curry sauce.

- **With Naan:** Pair with warm naan bread for a more substantial meal.

Spaghetti Squash Bolognese

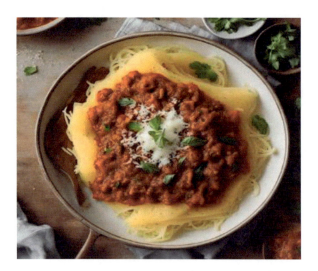

Spaghetti squash is a low-carb alternative to pasta, offering a light and nutritious base for this hearty Bolognese sauce. The rich, meaty sauce complements the tender squash strands, making it a satisfying dinner option.

Ingredients

- 1 large spaghetti squash
- 1 pound ground beef or turkey
- 1 onion, diced
- 2 garlic cloves, minced
- 1 carrot, grated
- 1 celery stalk, diced
- 1 can (14.5 ounces) crushed tomatoes
- 1/4 cup tomato paste
- 1 teaspoon dried oregano
- 1 teaspoon dried basil
- 1/2 cup beef or chicken broth
- 2 tablespoons olive oil
- Salt and pepper to taste
- Fresh parsley or basil for garnish

Instructions

1. **Cook the Spaghetti Squash:** Preheat your oven to 400°F (200°C). Cut the spaghetti squash in half lengthwise and remove the seeds. Drizzle with olive oil, season with salt and pepper, and place cut-side on a baking sheet. Roast for 40-45 minutes until the squash is tender and easily shredded with a fork.

2. **Make the Bolognese Sauce:** Heat olive oil in a large skillet over medium heat while the squash is roasting. Add the ground beef or turkey and cook until browned. Add the diced onion, garlic, carrot, celery, and sauté until softened.

3. **Simmer the Sauce:** Stir in the crushed tomatoes, tomato paste, oregano, basil, and broth—season with salt and pepper. Simmer for 20-30 minutes, allowing the flavors to meld.

4. **Serve:** Once the squash is cooked, use a fork to scrape out the strands of squash into a serving dish. Top with the Bolognese sauce and garnish with fresh parsley or basil.

Chef's Tips

- **Spaghetti Squash:** To make cutting easier, microwave the squash for a few minutes to soften the skin before slicing.

- **Sauce Variations:** Add a splash of red wine during the simmering process for a more decadent sauce.

Nutritional Information:

Calories: 350 | Protein: 25g | Total Fat: 18g | Saturated Fat: 6g | Cholesterol: 80mg | Sodium: 600mg | Fiber: 6g

Serving

- **With Cheese:** Top with grated Parmesan or mozzarella cheese for added richness.

- **As a Casserole:** Combine the squash and sauce in a baking dish, top with cheese, and bake for a few minutes until bubbly.

Grilled Chicken with Avocado Salsa

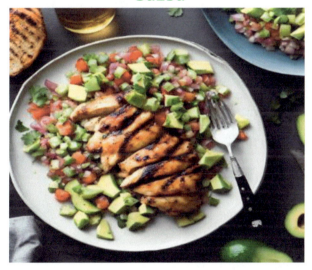

This grilled chicken dish is a light, refreshing dinner option with a vibrant avocado salsa. The combination of juicy chicken and creamy avocado makes it both satisfying and nutritious.

Ingredients

- 4 boneless, skinless chicken breasts

- 2 tablespoons olive oil

- 1 teaspoon ground cumin

- 1 teaspoon paprika

- 1 teaspoon garlic powder

- Salt and pepper to taste

- 2 ripe avocados, diced

- 1/2 red onion, finely chopped

- 1 jalapeño, seeded and minced

- 1/4 cup fresh cilantro, chopped

- Juice of 1 lime

Instructions

1. **Prepare the Chicken:** Preheat your grill to medium-high heat. Mix the olive oil, cumin, paprika, garlic powder, salt, and pepper in a small bowl. Rub the mixture over the chicken breasts.

2. **Grill the Chicken:** Grill the chicken for 6-7 minutes per side or until the internal temperature reaches 165°F (74°C). Remove from the grill and let rest.

3. **Make the Avocado Salsa:** In a medium bowl, combine the diced avocado, red onion, jalapeño, cilantro, and lime juice—season with salt and pepper to taste.

4. **Serve:** Serve the grilled chicken topped with avocado salsa.

Chef's Tips

- **Marinating Option:** For extra flavor, marinate the chicken in the spice mixture for 30 minutes before grilling.

- **Salsa Variations:** Add diced tomatoes or mango to the salsa for a sweeter twist.

Nutritional Information

Serving

- **With Rice:** Serve with a side of cilantro-lime rice or cauliflower rice.

- **With Salad:** Pair with a simple green salad or grilled vegetables for a balanced meal.

Beef Stroganoff with Creamy Coconut Milk Sauce

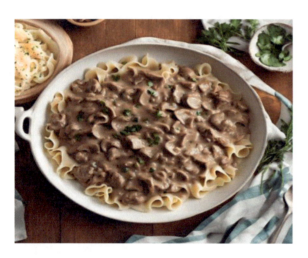

This beef stroganoff is a dairy-free version of the classic dish, made with tender beef strips in a rich coconut milk sauce. The creamy sauce pairs beautifully with the savory beef, making it a comforting and satisfying dinner.

Ingredients

- 1 pound beef sirloin or tenderloin sliced into thin strips

- 2 tablespoons coconut oil

- 1 onion, diced

- 2 garlic cloves, minced

- 8 ounces mushrooms, sliced

- 1 teaspoon paprika

- 1 tablespoon Dijon mustard

- 1 can (14 ounces) coconut milk

- 1/2 cup beef broth

- Salt and pepper to taste

- Fresh parsley, chopped (for garnish)

Instructions

1. **Cook the Beef:** Heat the coconut oil in a large skillet over medium-high heat. Add the beef strips and cook until browned on all sides. Remove the beef from the skillet and set aside.

2. **Cook the Vegetables:** In the same skillet, add the diced onion, garlic, and mushrooms. Sauté until the onions are soft and the mushrooms are browned.

3. **Make the Sauce:** Stir in the paprika and Dijon mustard, then pour in the coconut milk and beef broth. Bring to a simmer, and cook for 5-7 minutes until the sauce thickens slightly.

4. **Combine and Serve:** Return the beef to the skillet and simmer for another 5 minutes until the meat is heated through—season with salt and pepper. Serve garnished with fresh parsley.

Chef's Tips

- **Thickening the Sauce:** If the sauce is too thin, simmer uncovered for a few extra minutes to thicken.

- **Dairy-Free Alternative:** Coconut milk provides a creamy texture without dairy, but you can substitute with heavy cream if preferred.

Nutritional Information

<mark>Calories: 500 | Protein: 30g | Total Fat: 35g | Saturated Fat: 25g | Cholesterol: 90mg | Sodium: 450mg | Fiber: 2g</mark>

Serving

- **With Noodles:** Serve over egg noodles or zucchini noodles for a complete meal.

- **With Rice:** Pair with steamed rice or cauliflower rice.

Stuffed Bell Peppers with Ground Beef and Cheese

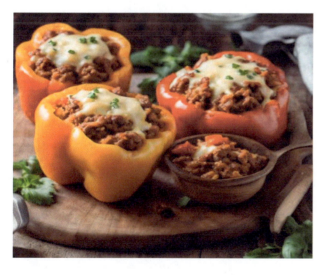

These stuffed bell peppers are a classic comfort food. Tender bell peppers are filled with a savory mixture of ground beef, cheese, and rice. It's a hearty and satisfying dinner option that's easy to prepare and flavorful.

Ingredients

- 4 large bell peppers, tops cut off and seeds removed
- 1 pound ground beef
- 1 cup cooked rice (white, brown, or cauliflower rice)
- 1 onion, diced
- 2 garlic cloves, minced
- 1 can (14.5 ounces) diced tomatoes, drained
- 1 teaspoon dried oregano
- 1 teaspoon dried basil
- 1 cup shredded cheese (cheddar, mozzarella, or a blend)
- 2 tablespoons olive oil
- Salt and pepper to taste
- Fresh parsley for garnish

Instructions

1. **Preheat the Oven:** Preheat your oven to 375°F (190°C). Lightly grease a baking dish with olive oil.

2. **Cook the Filling:** Heat the olive oil in a large skillet over medium heat. Add the ground beef, onion, and garlic, cooking until the meat is browned and the onion is soft. Stir in the cooked rice, diced tomatoes, oregano, basil, salt, and pepper.

3. **Stuff the Peppers:** Spoon the beef mixture into the prepared bell peppers, packing it tightly. Place the stuffed peppers in the baking dish.

4. **Bake:** Cover the dish with foil and bake for 30 minutes. Remove the foil, sprinkle the tops of the peppers with shredded cheese, and bake for an additional 10-15 minutes until the cheese is melted and bubbly.

5. **Serve:** Garnish with fresh parsley and serve warm.

Chef's Tips

- **Pepper Selection:** Choose bell peppers that are similar in size to ensure even cooking.

- **Cheese Options:** Experiment with different cheeses for varied flavors, such as Monterey Jack or Parmesan.

Nutritional Information

Calories: 450 | Protein: 30g | Total Fat: 25g | Saturated Fat: 10g | Cholesterol: 80mg | Sodium: 600mg | Fiber: 6g

Serving

- **With Salad:** Serve with a side salad or steamed vegetables.

- **With Sauce:** Top with a dollop of sour cream or marinara sauce for added richness.

Chapter 4

Snacks and Appetizers

Healthy Snacking Without Processed Oils

Snacking can be tricky for any diet, especially when avoiding processed oils and unhealthy ingredients. This chapter focuses on providing delicious snack and appetizer options made with wholesome, natural fats. These recipes are designed to satisfy you between meals without compromising your health. Whether you're looking for something crunchy, creamy, or savory, a snack here will hit the spot.

How to Satisfy Cravings the Right Way

Cravings are a natural part of eating, but it's essential to satisfy them in a way that supports your overall health goals. These snack and appetizer recipes are crafted to curb those cravings while providing vital nutrients. From nutrient-dense nuts and seeds to fresh vegetables paired with flavorful dips, these recipes will help you make intelligent snacking choices that align with your dietary needs.

Mixed Nuts Roasted in Coconut Oil

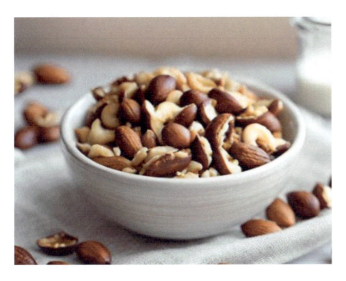

Mixed nuts roasted in coconut oil are a simple yet flavorful snack, perfect for satisfying hunger between meals. The coconut oil adds a subtle sweetness and enhances the natural flavors of the nuts, making them a delicious and nutritious option.

Ingredients

- 2 cups mixed raw nuts (such as almonds, cashews, pecans, and walnuts)
- 2 tablespoons coconut oil, melted
- 1 teaspoon sea salt
- 1/2 teaspoon ground cinnamon (optional)
- 1/4 teaspoon cayenne pepper (optional)

Instructions

1. **Preheat the Oven:** Preheat your oven to 350°F (175°C). Line a baking sheet with parchment paper.

2. **Prepare the Nuts:** In a large bowl, toss the mixed nuts with melted coconut oil, sea salt, cinnamon, and cayenne pepper (if using) until evenly coated.

3. **Roast the Nuts:** Spread the nuts in a single layer on the prepared baking sheet. Roast in the oven for 10-15 minutes, stirring halfway through, until the nuts are golden and fragrant.

4. **Cool and Serve:** Allow the nuts to cool completely before serving. Store any leftovers in an airtight container.

Chef's Tips

- **Flavor Variations:** Experiment with different spices for varied flavors, such as smoked paprika or rosemary.

- **Nut Selection:** Choose unsalted, raw nuts to control the amount of salt and ensure the freshest flavor.

Nutritional Information

Calories: 200 (per 1/4 cup serving) | Protein: 5g | Total Fat: 18g | Saturated Fat: 6g | Cholesterol: 0mg | Sodium: 150mg | Fiber: 3g

Serving

- **With Dried Fruit:** Mix with dried cranberries or raisins for a sweet and savory snack.

- **As a Topping:** Use as a topping for yogurt or salads for added crunch and flavor.

Guacamole with Homemade Almond Flour Chips

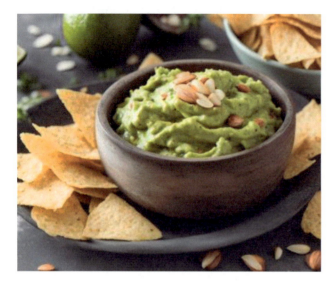

This guacamole is paired with homemade almond flour chips, a healthy, grain-free alternative to traditional tortilla chips. The combination is perfect for a satisfying snack or appetizer.

Ingredients for the Guacamole

- 3 ripe avocados, mashed
- Juice of 2 limes
- 1/2 cup diced tomatoes
- 1/4 cup finely chopped red onion
- 2 tablespoons fresh cilantro, chopped
- Salt and pepper to taste

- **For the Almond Flour Chips:**

- 1 1/2 cups almond flour
- 1/4 cup ground flaxseeds
- 1/4 teaspoon sea salt
- 1/4 cup water
- 1 tablespoon olive oil

Instructions

1. **Prepare the Guacamole:** In a medium bowl, mash the avocados until smooth. Stir in the lime juice, tomatoes, red onion, and cilantro—season with salt and pepper. Set aside.

2. **Make the Almond Flour Chips:** Preheat the oven to 350°F (175°C). Mix the almond flour, ground flaxseeds, and sea salt in a large bowl. Stir in the water and olive oil until a dough forms.

3. **Roll and Bake the Chips:** Place the dough between two sheets of parchment paper and roll it out to about 1/8-inch thickness. Remove the top sheet of parchment and cut the dough into triangles or squares. Transfer the dough, still on the parchment, to a baking sheet. Bake for 12-15 minutes until the chips are golden and crisp. Allow to cool before serving.

4. **Serve:** Serve the guacamole with the homemade almond flour chips.

Chef's Tips

- **Chip Thickness:** Roll the dough as evenly as possible to ensure uniform cooking.

- **Storage:** Store leftover chips in an airtight container to maintain crispness.

Nutritional Information

Calories: 350 (per serving with chips) | Protein: 8g | Total Fat: 30g | Saturated Fat: 4g | Cholesterol: 0mg | Sodium: 200mg | Fiber: 8g

Serving

- **With Salsa:** Serve alongside a fresh tomato salsa for additional dipping options.

- **As a salad topping,** crumble the chips over a salad for extra texture and flavor.

Full-fat cheese and Olive Platter

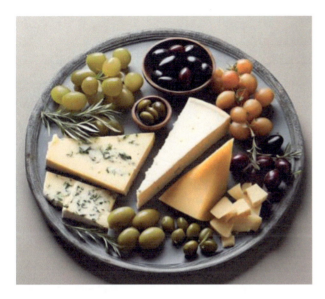

A simple yet elegant cheese and olive platter is an excellent snack or appetizer option. Featuring a variety of full-fat cheeses and marinated olives, this platter offers a rich, savory experience that's perfect for entertaining or enjoying as a snack.

Ingredients

- 8 ounces full-fat cheese (such as cheddar, gouda, brie, or blue cheese)

- 1 cup mixed olives (Kalamata, green, black, etc.)

- 1 tablespoon olive oil

- 1 tablespoon fresh herbs (such as rosemary or thyme)

- Crackers or sliced baguette (optional)

Instructions

1. **Prepare the Cheese:** Cut the cheese into bite-sized cubes or slices and arrange them on a serving platter.

2. **Marinate the Olives:** Toss the olives with olive oil and fresh herbs in a small bowl. Let them marinate for at least 15 minutes to absorb the flavors.

3. **Assemble the Platter:** Arrange the marinated olives around the cheese on the platter. Add crackers or sliced baguette if desired.

4. **Serve:** Serve the cheese and olive platter at room temperature.

Chef's Tips

- **Cheese Selection:** Include a variety of textures and flavors by choosing both hard and soft cheeses.

- **Olive Varieties:** Use a mix of different types of olives for a more interesting flavor profile.

Nutritional Information

Calories: 300 (per serving) | Protein: 12g | Total Fat: 25g | Saturated Fat: 12g | Cholesterol: 40mg | Sodium: 700mg | Fiber: 2g

Serving:

- **With Wine:** Pair with a glass of red or white wine for a more complete experience.

- **With Fruit:** Add fresh or dried fruit, such as grapes or figs, for a sweet contrast.

Spicy Roasted Chickpeas in Olive Oil

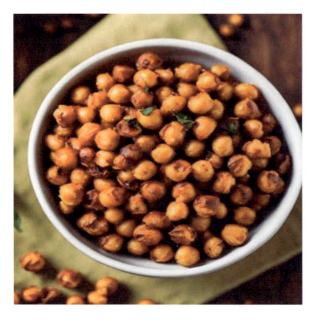

Spicy roasted chickpeas are a crunchy and satisfying snack. They offer a good source of protein and fiber. Tossed in olive oil and seasoned with spices, they make a great alternative to traditional salty snacks.

Ingredients

- 1 can (15 ounces) chickpeas, drained and rinsed
- 2 tablespoons olive oil
- 1 teaspoon smoked paprika
- 1/2 teaspoon ground cumin
- 1/4 teaspoon cayenne pepper
- Salt and pepper to taste

Instructions

1. **Preheat the Oven:** Preheat your oven to 400°F (200°C). Line a baking sheet with parchment paper.

2. **Prepare the Chickpeas:** Pat the Chickpeas dry with a paper towel to remove any excess moisture. This will help them crisp up in the oven.

3. **Season the Chickpeas:** In a large bowl, toss the chickpeas with olive oil, smoked paprika, cumin, cayenne pepper, salt, and pepper until evenly coated.

4. **Roast the Chickpeas:** Spread the chickpeas in a single layer on the prepared baking sheet. Roast for 25-30 minutes, shaking the pan halfway through, until the chickpeas are crispy and golden brown.

5. **Serve:** Allow the chickpeas to cool slightly before serving.

Chef's Tips

- **Crispiness:** Bake extra crispy chickpeas a bit longer, but watch closely to prevent burning.

- **Flavor Variations:** To change the flavor profile, experiment with different spices, such as curry powder or garlic powder.

Nutritional Information

Calories: 150 (per 1/4 cup serving) | Protein: 6g | Total Fat: 7g | Saturated Fat: 1g | Cholesterol: 0mg | Sodium: 250mg | Fiber: 6g

Serving

- **With Salad:** Add the roasted chickpeas to salads for a crunchy topping.

- **As a Snack:** Enjoy them as a healthy, portable snack.

Avocado Deviled Eggs

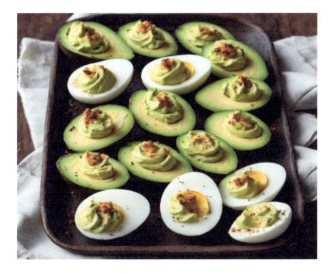

Avocado deviled eggs are a creamy and nutritious twist on the classic recipe. The addition of avocado adds healthy fats and a vibrant green color, making these deviled eggs delicious and visually appealing.

Ingredients

- 6 large eggs, hard-boiled and peeled

- 1 ripe avocado, pitted and mashed

- 1 tablespoon lime juice

- 1 tablespoon mayonnaise (optional)

- 1/2 teaspoon Dijon mustard

- Salt and pepper to taste

- Paprika, for garnish

- Fresh chives, chopped (for garnish)

Instructions

1. **Prepare the Eggs:** Cut the hard-boiled eggs in half lengthwise. Remove the yolks and place them in a bowl.

2. **Make the Filling:** Mash the egg yolks with the avocado, lime juice, mayonnaise (if using), Dijon mustard, salt, and pepper until smooth and creamy.

3. **Fill the Eggs:** Spoon or pipe the avocado mixture back into the egg white halves.

4. **Garnish and Serve:** Sprinkle the deviled eggs with paprika and chopped chives. Serve immediately or refrigerate until ready to serve.

Chef's Tips

- **Ripeness:** Use a ripe avocado for the creamiest texture.

- **Make Ahead:** These deviled eggs can be made a few hours ahead and stored in the refrigerator.

Nutritional Information

Calories: 120 (per 2 halves) | Protein: 6g | Total Fat: 10g | Saturated Fat: 2g | Cholesterol: 140mg | Sodium: 150mg | Fiber: 3g

Serving

- **With Veggies:** Serve alongside fresh veggie sticks for a complete snack.

- **As an Appetizer:** These deviled eggs make a great party appetizer or potluck dish.

Baked Kale Chips with Sea Salt

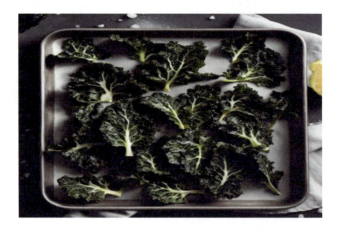

Baked kale chips are a crunchy, nutrient-dense snack that's easy to make and delicious. Seasoned simply with olive oil and sea salt, they are a healthy alternative to traditional potato chips, offering a satisfying crunch without the processed ingredients.

Ingredients

- 1 bunch of kale, stems removed and leaves torn into bite-sized pieces

- 2 tablespoons olive oil

- Sea salt, to taste

Instructions

1. **Preheat the Oven:** Preheat your oven to 300°F (150°C). Line a baking sheet with parchment paper.

2. **Prepare the Kale:** In a large bowl, toss the kale leaves with olive oil until evenly coated. Spread the kale in a single layer on the prepared baking sheet.

3. **Bake the Kale:** Bake for 20-25 minutes until the kale is crisp but not burnt. Keep an eye on them to ensure they don't overcook.

4. **Season and Serve:** Remove the kale chips from the oven and sprinkle with sea salt. Let them cool slightly before serving.

Chef's Tips

- **Even Coating:** Massage the olive oil into the kale leaves to ensure they are evenly coated and crisp up nicely.

- **Storage:** Store any leftover chips in an airtight container to maintain their crispness.

Nutritional Information:

Calories: 60 (per serving) | Protein: 2g | Total Fat: 5g | Saturated Fat: 1g | Cholesterol: 0mg | Sodium: 120mg | Fiber: 2g

Serving:

- **With Dip:** Serve with a healthy dip like hummus or guacamole.

- **As a Topping,** Crumble over salads or soups for added texture.

Coconut Macaroons with Dark Chocolate Drizzle

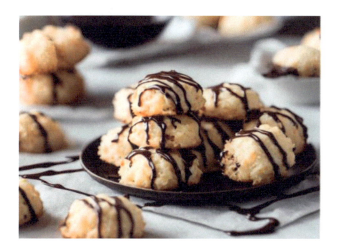

These coconut macaroons are an indulgent and relatively healthy sweet treat. Made with shredded coconut and drizzled with dark chocolate, they're perfect for satisfying a sweet tooth without the guilt.

Ingredients

- 2 cups unsweetened shredded coconut
- 1/2 cup almond flour
- 1/4 cup honey or maple syrup
- 2 egg whites
- 1/2 teaspoon vanilla extract
- 1/4 teaspoon sea salt
- 1/4 cup dark chocolate, melted

Instructions

1. **Preheat the Oven:** Preheat your oven to 350°F (175°C). Line a baking sheet with parchment paper.

2. **Mix the Ingredients:** In a large bowl, combine the shredded coconut, almond flour, honey, egg whites, vanilla extract, and sea salt. Mix until well combined.

3. **Form the Macaroons:** Using a tablespoon, scoop the mixture and shape it into small mounds. Place them on the prepared baking sheet.

4. **Bake:** Bake for 15-20 minutes until the edges are golden brown. Let the macaroons cool completely on a wire rack.

5. **Drizzle with Chocolate:** Drizzle the macaroons with melted dark chocolate once cooled. Allow the chocolate to set before serving.

Chef's Tips

- **Chocolate Quality:** Use dark chocolate with at least 70% cocoa for the best flavor and health benefits.

- **Storage:** Store in an airtight container at room temperature for up to a week.

Nutritional Information

Calories: 120 (per macaroon) | Protein: 2g | Total Fat: 9g | Saturated Fat: 7g | Cholesterol: 0mg | Sodium: 50mg | Fiber: 3g

Serving

- **With Coffee:** Pair with a cup of coffee or tea for a delightful snack.

- **As a Dessert:** Serve as a light dessert at the end of a meal.

Bacon-Wrapped Jalapeño Poppers

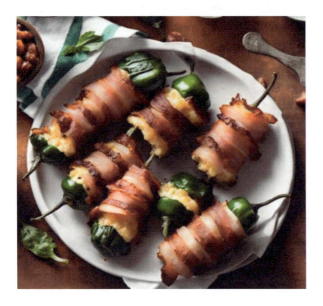

Bacon-wrapped jalapeño poppers are a spicy, savory snack for parties or game days. The combination of crispy bacon, creamy cheese, and spicy jalapeños makes for an irresistible appetizer.

Ingredients

- 8 large jalapeños, halved and seeded
- 4 ounces cream cheese, softened
- 1/2 cup shredded cheddar cheese
- 8 slices bacon, cut in half
- 1/4 teaspoon garlic powder
- 1/4 teaspoon smoked paprika
- Toothpicks (optional)

Instructions

1. **Preheat the Oven:** Preheat your oven to 400°F (200°C). Line a baking sheet with parchment paper.

2. **Prepare the Filling:** In a small bowl, mix the cream cheese, shredded cheddar cheese, garlic powder, and smoked paprika until well combined.

3. **Stuff the Jalapeños:** Spoon the cheese mixture into each jalapeño half, filling them generously.

4. **Wrap with Bacon:** Wrap each stuffed jalapeño with a half slice of bacon, securing with a toothpick if needed. Place the jalapeños on the prepared baking sheet.

5. **Bake:** Bake for 20-25 minutes until the bacon is crispy and the cheese is bubbly.

6. **Serve:** Let the poppers cool slightly before serving.

Chef's Tips

- **Spice Level:** For milder poppers, use smaller, less mature jalapeños or remove more seeds and membranes.

- **Bacon Variety:** Use thin-sliced bacon for easier wrapping and quicker cooking.

Nutritional Information:

Calories: 100 (per popper) | Protein: 5g | Total Fat: 8g | Saturated Fat: 3g | Cholesterol: 15mg | Sodium: 250mg | Fiber: 1g

Serving:

- **With Dip:** Serve with ranch dressing or sour cream for dipping.

- **As an Appetizer,** These poppers make an excellent starter for any gathering or casual meal.

Almond Butter Stuffed Dates

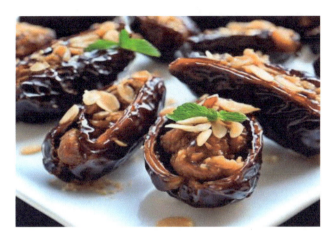

Almond butter stuffed dates are a sweet and satisfying snack, combining the natural sweetness of dates with the rich, nutty flavor of almond butter. They're simple to make and perfect for a quick energy boost.

Ingredients

- 12 Medjool dates, pitted
- 1/4 cup almond butter
- 1/4 cup chopped nuts (such as almonds, walnuts, or pistachios)
- 1/4 teaspoon sea salt

Instructions

1. **Prepare the Dates:** Carefully slit each date lengthwise and remove the pit if not already pitted.

2. **Stuff the Dates:** Spoon about 1 teaspoon of almond butter into the cavity of each date.

3. **Add Toppings:** Sprinkle the stuffed dates with chopped nuts and a pinch of sea salt.

4. **Serve:** Serve immediately or store in the refrigerator until ready to enjoy.

Chef's Tips

- **Nut Butter Options:** Substitute almond butter with peanut butter, cashew butter, or any other nut butter you choose.

- **Sweetness Level:** Drizzle the dates with a bit of honey or maple syrup for a sweeter treat.

Nutritional Information

Calories: 90 (per date) | Protein: 2g | Total Fat: 4g | Saturated Fat: 0.5g | Cholesterol: 0mg | Sodium: 20mg | Fiber: 2g

Serving

- **With Coffee:** Enjoy with a cup of coffee or tea for a sweet snack.

- **As a Dessert:** Serve as a light and healthy dessert option.

Cream Cheese and Smoked Salmon Bites

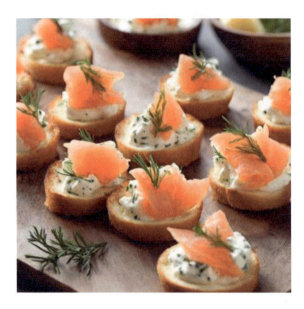

These cream cheese and smoked salmon bites are an elegant and flavorful appetizer, perfect for entertaining. The combination of creamy cheese, savory smoked salmon, and fresh herbs are sure to impress your guests.

Ingredients

- 8 ounces cream cheese, softened

- 4 ounces smoked salmon, thinly sliced

- 1 tablespoon fresh dill, chopped

- 1 tablespoon capers, drained

- 1 tablespoon lemon juice

- 1 cucumber, sliced into rounds

Instructions:

1. **Prepare the Cream Cheese:** In a small bowl, mix the cream cheese with lemon juice and chopped dill until smooth.

2. **Assemble the Bites:** Spread a small amount of the cream cheese mixture onto each cucumber slice. Top with a piece of smoked salmon and a few capers.

3. **Garnish and Serve:** Garnish with additional dill if desired, and serve immediately.

Chef's Tips

- **Cucumber Slices:** Use a mandoline for even, thin cucumber slices.

- **Salmon Selection:** Choose high-quality smoked salmon for the best flavor.

Nutritional Information

Calories: 50 (per bite) | Protein: 3g | Total Fat: 4g | Saturated Fat: 2g | Cholesterol: 15mg | Sodium: 150mg | Fiber: 0g

Serving

- **With Crackers:** Serve alongside crackers or crostini for a more substantial appetizer.

- **As a Canapé:** These bites make an elegant canapé for a cocktail party or holiday gathering.

Cucumber Slices with Cream Cheese and Herbs

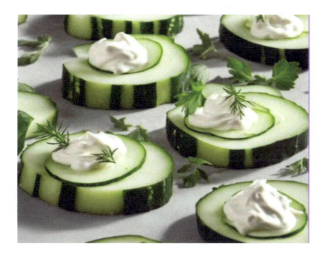

Cucumber slices with cream cheese and herbs are a light, refreshing appetizer perfect for any occasion. The cool, crisp cucumber pairs beautifully with the rich, creamy cheese, making it a delightful snack or starter.

Ingredients

- 1 large cucumber, sliced into rounds

- 8 ounces cream cheese, softened

- 1 tablespoon fresh chives, chopped

- 1 tablespoon fresh parsley, chopped

- 1 tablespoon lemon juice

- Salt and pepper to taste

Instructions

1. **Prepare the Cream Cheese:** In a small bowl, mix the cream cheese with lemon juice, chopped chives, and parsley until smooth—season with salt and pepper to taste.

2. **Assemble the Bites:** Spread the cream cheese mixture onto each cucumber slice.

3. **Garnish and Serve:** Garnish with additional herbs or a sprinkle of lemon zest. Serve immediately.

Chef's Tips

- **Herb Variations:** Experiment with different herbs, such as dill or basil, for varied flavors.

- **Make Ahead:** Prepare the cream cheese mixture and store it in the refrigerator until ready to assemble.

Nutritional Information

Calories: 40 (per slice) | Protein: 1g | Total Fat: 4g | Saturated Fat: 2g | Cholesterol: 10mg | Sodium: 50mg | Fiber: 0g

Serving

- **With Crackers:** Serve with crackers or breadsticks for added texture.

- **As a Light Snack:** Enjoy a refreshing and healthy snack anytime.

Deviled Ham Spread with Almond Crackers

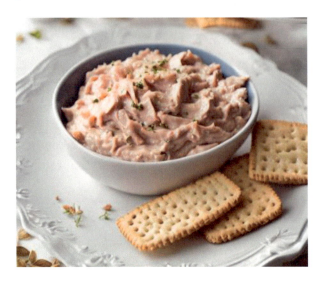

This deviled ham spread is a savory and creamy appetizer, perfect for spreading on almond crackers. Made with cooked ham, cream cheese, and spices, it's a flavorful and satisfying snack that's great for gatherings or as a quick snack.

Ingredients

- 1 cup cooked ham, finely chopped

- 4 ounces cream cheese, softened

- 2 tablespoons Dijon mustard

- 1 tablespoon mayonnaise

- 1 teaspoon Worcestershire sauce

- 1/4 teaspoon smoked paprika

- Salt and pepper to taste

- Almond crackers for serving

Instructions

1. **Prepare the Spread:** In a medium bowl, mix the chopped ham, cream cheese, Dijon mustard, mayonnaise, Worcestershire sauce, smoked paprika, salt, and pepper until well combined.

2. **Chill the Spread:** Cover the bowl and refrigerate the spread for at least 30 minutes to allow the flavors to meld.

3. **Serve:** Serve the deviled ham spread with almond crackers.

Chef's Tips

- **Texture:** Blend the ingredients in a food processor until the desired consistency is reached for a smoother spread.

- **Flavor Adjustments:** Adjust the seasoning to taste, adding more mustard or paprika for extra flavor.

Nutritional Information

Calories: 100 (per serving with crackers) | Protein: 5g | Total Fat: 8g | Saturated Fat: 3g | Cholesterol: 25mg | Sodium: 350mg | Fiber: 1g

Serving

- **With Vegetables:** Serve with sliced cucumbers or celery sticks for a low-carb option.

- **As a Sandwich Spread:** Use the deviled ham spread to fill sandwiches or wraps.

Eggplant Dip with Fresh Vegetables

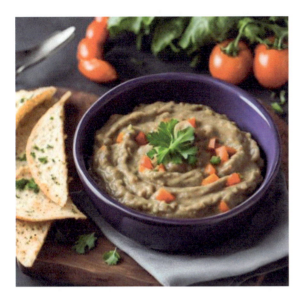

This eggplant dip, or baba ganoush, is a smoky, creamy appetizer made with roasted eggplant, tahini, and garlic. It's a healthy and flavorful snack paired with fresh vegetables, perfect for any occasion.

Ingredients

- 2 large eggplants
- 1/4 cup tahini
- 2 garlic cloves, minced
- Juice of 1 lemon
- 2 tablespoons olive oil
- 1/2 teaspoon ground cumin
- Salt and pepper to taste
- Fresh vegetables (carrot sticks, cucumber slices, bell pepper strips) for dipping

Instructions

1. **Roast the Eggplant:** Preheat your oven to 400°F (200°C). Prick the eggplants with a fork and place them on a baking sheet. Roast 30-40 minutes until the eggplants are soft and the skins are charred. Allow to cool slightly.

2. **Make the Dip:** Once cooled, scoop the flesh of the eggplants into a food processor. Add the tahini, garlic, lemon juice, olive oil, cumin, salt, and pepper. Blend until smooth and creamy.

3. **Serve:** Transfer the dip to a serving bowl and drizzle with extra olive oil. Serve with fresh vegetables.

Chef's Tips

- **Smokiness:** Grill the eggplants over an open flame instead of roasting them in the oven for an extra smoky flavor.

- **Consistency:** If the dip is too thick, add a little water or more lemon juice to reach your desired consistency.

Nutritional Information

Calories: 80 (per serving) | Protein: 2g | Total Fat: 6g | Saturated Fat: 1g | Cholesterol: 0mg | Sodium: 150mg | Fiber: 4g

Serving:

- **With Pita:** Serve with toasted pita bread or chips for a more traditional pairing.

- **As a Spread:** Use the eggplant dip as a spread for sandwiches or wraps.

Marinated Artichokes and Olives

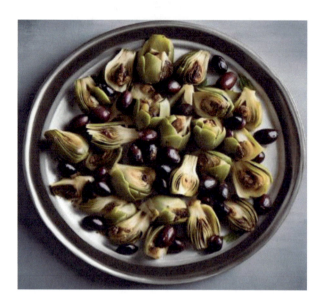

Marinated artichokes and olives are a savory and tangy appetizer that's easy to prepare and flavorful. The combination of tender artichoke hearts and briny olives makes a delicious snack perfect for entertaining or enjoying with a glass of wine.

Ingredients

- 1 jar (14 ounces) marinated artichoke hearts, drained
- 1 cup mixed olives (Kalamata, green, black, etc.)
- 2 tablespoons olive oil
- 1 tablespoon red wine vinegar
- 1 garlic clove, minced
- 1 teaspoon dried oregano
- 1/2 teaspoon crushed red pepper flakes (optional)
- Fresh parsley, chopped (for garnish)

Instructions

1. **Prepare the Marinade:** In a large bowl, whisk together the olive oil, red wine vinegar, minced garlic, oregano, and red pepper flakes.

2. **Marinate the Artichokes and Olives:** Add the drained artichoke hearts and mixed olives to the bowl. Toss to coat evenly with the marinade. Cover and refrigerate for at least 1 hour to allow the flavors to meld.

3. **Serve:** Transfer the marinated artichokes and olives to a serving dish. Garnish with chopped parsley and serve.

Chef's Tips

- **Marinating Time:** The longer the artichokes and olives marinate, the more flavorful they will become. Prepare them a day ahead for the best results.

- **Olive Variety:** Use a mix of different types of olives for a more complex flavor profile.

Nutritional Information

Calories: 100 (per serving) | Protein: 1g | Total Fat: 9g | Saturated Fat: 1g | Cholesterol: 0mg | Sodium: 350mg | Fiber: 3g

Serving

- **With Bread:** Serve with slices of crusty bread or crackers.

- **As an Antipasto:** Include meats, cheeses, and roasted vegetables as part of an antipasto platter.

Chapter 5

Sauces and Dressings

Enhancing Flavor with Natural Ingredients

Sauces and dressings are the key to elevating the flavors of your meals, turning simple dishes into something extraordinary. Using natural, wholesome ingredients, you can create delicious sauces and dressings that enhance the taste and contribute to your overall health. This chapter is dedicated to providing recipes free from processed oils and additives, ensuring that each bite is as nutritious as flavorful.

Homemade Alternatives to Store-Bought Products

Many store-bought sauces and dressings contain unhealthy oils, preservatives, and sugars that can detract from the nutritional value of your meals. Making your sauces and dressings at home allows you to control the ingredients, ensuring you only consume what's best for your body. In this chapter, you'll find various recipes that are easy to prepare, versatile, and perfect for adding that extra flavor to your favorite dishes.

Classic Hollandaise Sauce with Grass-Fed Butter

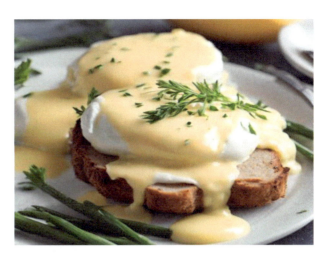

Hollandaise sauce is a rich and creamy sauce made with egg yolks, lemon juice, and butter. This version uses grass-fed butter, which adds a deeper flavor and provides beneficial nutrients. It's perfect for drizzling over eggs, vegetables, or fish.

Ingredients

- 3 large egg yolks

- 1 tablespoon lemon juice

- 1/2 cup grass-fed butter, melted and warm

- 1/4 teaspoon sea salt

- Pinch of cayenne pepper (optional)

Instructions

1. **Whisk the Egg Yolks:** In a heatproof bowl, whisk the egg yolks and lemon juice together until they are light and frothy.

2. **Cook the Sauce:** Place the bowl over a pot of simmering water (double boiler method). Continue whisking the egg yolk mixture constantly.

3. **Add the Butter:** Slowly drizzle in the melted butter while whisking continuously. The sauce should thicken as the butter is incorporated. Be careful not to overheat, which can cause the eggs to scramble.

4. **Season and Serve:** Once the sauce has thickened, remove it from the heat. Stir in the sea salt and cayenne pepper, if using. Serve immediately.

Chef's Tips

- **Temperature Control:** Keep the heat low to prevent the eggs from scrambling. Remove the sauce from the heat and whisk briskly if the sauce thickens too quickly.

- **Make Ahead:** Hollandaise sauce is best served fresh, but you can keep it warm in a thermos for up to 30 minutes.

Nutritional Information

Calories: 200 (per serving) | Protein: 2g | Total Fat: 22g | Saturated Fat: 14g | Cholesterol: 145mg | Sodium: 120mg | Fiber: 0g

Serving

- **With Eggs Benedict:** Serve over poached eggs for classic Eggs Benedict.

- **With Vegetables:** Drizzle over steamed asparagus or roasted broccoli for a rich, indulgent side dish.

Olive Oil and Balsamic Vinaigrette

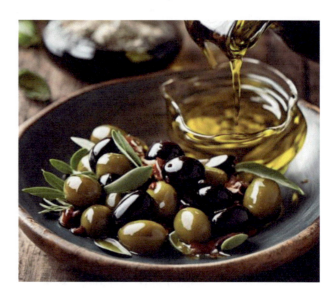

This olive oil and balsamic vinaigrette is a simple, classic dressing perfect for salads, roasted vegetables, or marinade. Combining extra virgin olive oil and balsamic vinegar creates a balanced and flavorful dressing that's easy to make and versatile.

Ingredients

- 1/4 cup extra virgin olive oil

- 2 tablespoons balsamic vinegar

- 1 teaspoon Dijon mustard

- 1 garlic clove, minced

- 1 teaspoon honey (optional)

- Salt and pepper to taste

Instructions

1. **Mix the Ingredients:** In a small bowl, whisk together the balsamic vinegar, Dijon mustard, minced garlic, and honey (if using).

2. **Emulsify the Dressing:** Slowly drizzle in the olive oil while whisking continuously to emulsify the dressing.

3. **Season and Serve:** Season with salt and pepper to taste. Serve over salads or use as a marinade.

Chef's Tips

- **Honey Addition:** The honey helps to balance the acidity of the vinegar, but it can be omitted if you prefer a sharper flavor.

- **Storage:** Leftover vinaigrette can be stored in a sealed container in the refrigerator for up to a week. Shake well before using.

Nutritional Information

Calories: 120 (per tablespoon) | Protein: 0g | Total Fat: 14g | Saturated Fat: 2g | Cholesterol: 0mg | Sodium: 20mg | Fiber: 0g

Serving

- **With Salad:** Use as a dressing for mixed greens or a Caprese salad.

- **As a Marinade:** Marinate chicken or beef before grilling for added flavor.

Coconut Milk Ranch Dressing

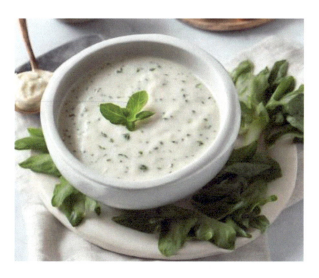

This coconut milk ranch dressing is a dairy-free alternative to traditional ranch. Its creamy base is coconut milk. It's perfect for salads, dipping vegetables, or drizzling over-baked potatoes.

Ingredients

- 1/2 cup coconut milk (full-fat, canned)

- 1/4 cup mayonnaise (preferably homemade)

- 1 tablespoon apple cider vinegar

- 1 garlic clove, minced

- 1 tablespoon fresh dill, chopped

- 1 tablespoon fresh parsley, chopped

- 1 teaspoon onion powder

- Salt and pepper to taste

Instructions

1. **Combine Ingredients:** In a medium bowl, whisk together the coconut milk, mayonnaise, and apple cider vinegar until smooth.

2. **Add Herbs and Seasoning:** Mix the minced garlic, dill, parsley, onion powder, salt, and pepper.

3. **Chill and Serve:** Refrigerate the dressing for at least 30 minutes to allow the flavors to meld. Serve cold.

Chef's Tips

- **Consistency:** If the dressing is too thick, thin it with more coconut milk or water.

- **Herb Options:** Feel free to experiment with fresh herbs like chives, basil, or cilantro.

Nutritional Information

Calories: 90 (per tablespoon) | Protein: 0g | Total Fat: 9g | Saturated Fat: 6g | Cholesterol: 5mg | Sodium: 60mg | Fiber: 0g

Serving:

- **With Salad:** Use as a creamy dressing for green salads or coleslaw.

- **As a Dip:** Serve for raw vegetables or chicken wings.

Ghee Garlic Sauce

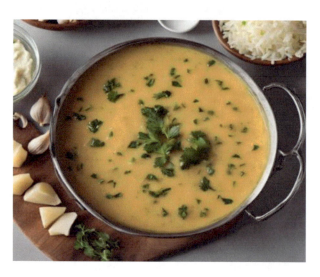

This ghee garlic sauce is a rich, flavorful addition to meats, vegetables, or grains. Made with clarified butter (ghee) and fresh garlic, it adds a depth of flavor to any dish and is particularly significant for those following a ketogenic or paleo diet.

Ingredients

- 1/4 cup ghee

- 4 garlic cloves, minced

- 1 tablespoon lemon juice

- 1 tablespoon fresh parsley, chopped (optional)

- Salt to taste

Instructions

1. **Melt the Ghee:** In a small saucepan, melt the ghee over medium heat.

2. **Cook the Garlic:** Add the minced garlic to the melted ghee and sauté for 2-3 minutes, until the garlic is fragrant and lightly golden.

3. **To finish the Sauce,** Stir in the lemon juice and salt. Remove from heat and stir in the fresh parsley if using.

4. **Serve:** Serve warm over your favorite dishes.

Chef's Tips

- **Garlic Flavor:** For a more intense garlic flavor, cook it on low heat for a more extended period, allowing it to infuse the ghee fully.

- **Versatility:** This sauce can also be used as a dip for bread or drizzled over pasta.

Nutritional Information

Calories: 110 (per tablespoon) | Protein: 0g | Total Fat: 12g | Saturated Fat: 7g | Cholesterol: 30mg | Sodium: 60mg | Fiber: 0g

Serving

- **With Meat:** Drizzle over grilled steaks or roasted chicken for added richness.

- **With Vegetables:** Toss with roasted or steamed vegetables for a flavorful side dish.

Avocado Oil Mayonnaise

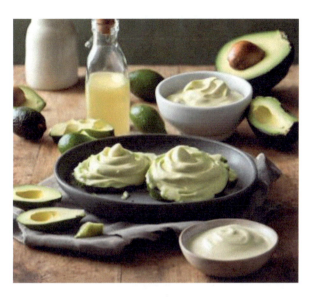

Avocado oil mayonnaise is a healthier alternative to traditional mayonnaise, made with nutrient-rich avocado oil. It's creamy, smooth, and perfect for spreading on sandwiches, mixing into salads, or using as a dip.

Ingredients

- 1 large egg (at room temperature)

- 1 tablespoon Dijon mustard

- 1 tablespoon lemon juice

- 1 cup avocado oil

- Salt to taste

Instructions

1. **Combine Ingredients:** Add the egg, Dijon mustard, and lemon juice to a tall, narrow container.

2. **Emulsify the Mayonnaise:** Using an immersion blender, blend the ingredients while slowly pour in the avocado oil. Continue mixing until the mixture thickens into mayonnaise.

3. **Season and Store:** Season with salt to taste. Store in an airtight container in the refrigerator for up to a week.

Chef's Tips

- **Blending Method:** If you don't have an immersion blender, you can use a regular blender or food processor. Be sure to add the oil very slowly to ensure proper emulsification.

- **Flavor Variations:** Add garlic, herbs, or spices to create flavored mayonnaise.

Nutritional Information

Calories: 100 (per tablespoon) | Protein: 0g | Total Fat: 11g | Saturated Fat: 1.5g | Cholesterol: 10mg | Sodium: 40mg | Fiber: 0g

Serving

- **With Sandwiches:** Spread on sandwiches or wraps for a creamy addition.

- **As a Dip:** Use as a base for dipping sauces or mix into potato or egg salads.

Lemon Tahini Dressing

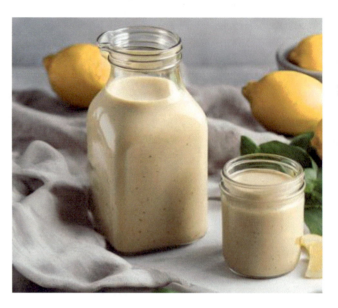

This lemon tahini dressing is creamy and tangy, perfect for drizzling over salads, roasted vegetables, or grains. Tahini and lemon juice combine to create a balanced flavor profile that adds freshness to any dish.

Ingredients

- 1/4 cup tahini

- 2 tablespoons lemon juice (about 1 lemon)

- 2 tablespoons water

- 1 garlic clove, minced

- 1 tablespoon extra-virgin olive oil

- 1 teaspoon maple syrup (optional)

- Salt and pepper to taste

Instructions

1. **Mix the Ingredients:** In a medium bowl, whisk together the tahini, lemon juice, water, minced garlic, and olive oil until smooth.

2. **Adjust Consistency:** If the dressing is too thick, add one tablespoon more water until it reaches your desired consistency.

3. **Season and Serve:** Stir in the maple syrup (if using), and season with salt and pepper to taste. Serve immediately or store in the refrigerator.

Chef's Tips

- **Consistency Control:** Tahini can vary in thickness, so adjust the water amount to achieve your preferred consistency.

- **Storage:** This dressing can be stored in the refrigerator for up to a week. Stir before using as it may thicken when chilled.

Nutritional Information

Calories: 80 (per tablespoon) | Protein: 2g | Total Fat: 7g | Saturated Fat: 1g | Cholesterol: 0mg | Sodium: 20mg | Fiber: 1g

Serving

- **With Salads:** Drizzle over a simple green salad or a grain bowl.

- **With Vegetables:** Use as a dipping sauce for raw or roasted vegetables.

Homemade Pesto with Olive Oil

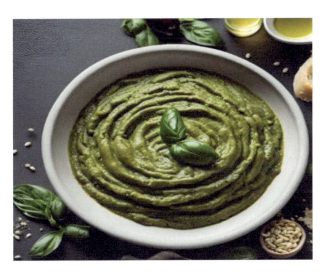

This homemade pesto is a vibrant and flavorful sauce made with fresh basil, garlic, pine nuts, and extra virgin olive oil. It's perfect for tossing with pasta, spreading on sandwiches, or using as a marinade.

Ingredients

- 2 cups fresh basil leaves, packed

- 1/4 cup pine nuts (or walnuts)

- 2 garlic cloves

- 1/2 cup extra virgin olive oil

- 1/2 cup grated Parmesan cheese

- Salt and pepper to taste

- Juice of 1/2 lemon (optional)

Instructions

1. **Blend the Ingredients:** In a food processor, combine the basil leaves, pine nuts, and garlic. Pulse until coarsely chopped.

2. **Add the Olive Oil:** With the food processor running, slowly drizzle in the olive oil until the mixture is smooth.

3. **To finish the Pesto,** Stir in the grated Parmesan cheese and season with salt and pepper. If desired, add lemon juice for a touch of brightness.

4. **Serve:** Use immediately or store in an airtight container in the refrigerator.

Chef's Tips

- **Nuts Substitution:** Pine nuts can be expensive; feel free to substitute with walnuts, almonds, or sunflower seeds.

- **Storage:** Pesto can be stored in the refrigerator for up to a week or frozen in ice cube trays for extended storage.

Nutritional Information

Calories: 90 (per tablespoon) | Protein: 2g | Total Fat: 9g | Saturated Fat: 2g | Cholesterol: 4mg | Sodium: 70mg | Fiber: 1g

Serving

- **With Pasta:** Toss with your favorite pasta or zoodles for a quick meal.

- **As a Spread:** Spread on sandwiches, wraps, or use as a base for pizza.

Chipotle Aioli with Avocado Oil

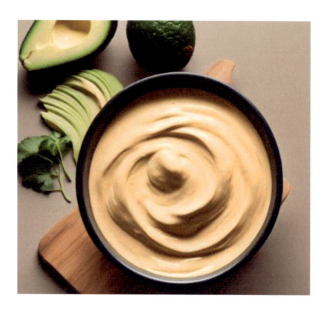

Chipotle aioli is a smoky, spicy sauce made with chipotle peppers, garlic, and creamy avocado oil mayonnaise. It's perfect for spreading on sandwiches and burgers or using as a dip for fries and veggies.

Ingredients

- 1/2 cup avocado oil mayonnaise (homemade or store-bought)

- 1 chipotle pepper in adobo sauce, minced

- 1 garlic clove, minced

- 1 tablespoon lime juice

- Salt and pepper to taste

Instructions

1. **Mix the Ingredients:** In a small bowl, whisk together the avocado oil mayonnaise, minced chipotle pepper, garlic, and lime juice until smooth.

2. **Season and Serve:** Season with salt and pepper to taste. Serve immediately or refrigerate until ready to use.

Chef's Tips

- **Heat Level:** Adjust the amount of chipotle pepper to your preferred heat level. For a milder sauce, use half a pepper or remove the seeds.

- **Storage:** Store in an airtight container in the refrigerator for up to a week.

Nutritional Information

Calories: 100 (per tablespoon) | Protein: 0g | Total Fat: 11g | Saturated Fat: 1.5g | Cholesterol: 10mg | Sodium: 80mg | Fiber: 0g

Serving

- **With Tacos:** Drizzle over tacos or fajitas for added flavor.

- **As a Dip:** Serve for sweet potato fries or grilled vegetables.

Chimichurri Sauce with Fresh Herbs

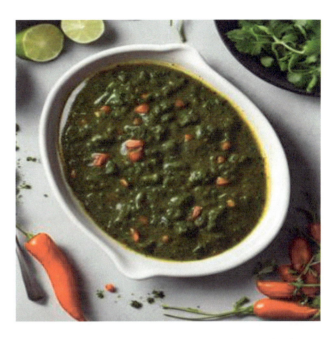

Chimichurri is a bright, tangy sauce with fresh herbs, garlic, and vinegar. Originally from Argentina, it's typically served with grilled meats but is also delicious on vegetables, fish, or as a marinade.

Ingredients

- 1 cup fresh parsley, finely chopped

- 1/2 cup fresh cilantro, finely chopped

- 4 garlic cloves, minced

- 2 tablespoons red wine vinegar

- 1/2 cup extra virgin olive oil

- 1 teaspoon dried oregano

- 1/2 teaspoon crushed red pepper flakes (optional)

- Salt and pepper to taste

Instructions

1. **Combine the Herbs:** In a medium bowl, mix the chopped parsley, cilantro, garlic, oregano, and red pepper flakes.

2. **Add the Vinegar and Oil:** Stir in the red wine vinegar, then slowly drizzle in the olive oil, mixing until well combined.

3. **Season and Serve:** Season with salt and pepper to taste. Serve immediately, or let it sit for an hour to develop the flavors.

Chef's Tips

- **Freshness:** Chimichurri is best made with fresh herbs. Avoid using dried herbs, which won't provide the same bright flavor.

- **Storage:** Store in the refrigerator for up to a week. Bring to room temperature before serving.

Nutritional Information

Calories: 90 (per tablespoon) | Protein: 0g | Total Fat: 9g | Saturated Fat: 1.5g | Cholesterol: 0mg | Sodium: 10mg | Fiber: 0g

Serving:

- **With Grilled Meats:** Serve over grilled steak, chicken, or pork.

- **As a Marinade:** Use a marinade for meats or vegetables before grilling.

Almond Butter Satay Sauce

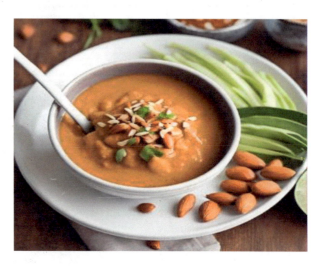

This almond butter satay sauce is a nutty, savory sauce with a touch of sweetness and spice. It's a delicious accompaniment to grilled chicken, beef, or tofu and also works well as a dipping sauce for vegetables or spring rolls.

Ingredients

- 1/4 cup almond butter

- 1/4 cup coconut milk

- 1 tablespoon soy sauce or tamari

- 1 tablespoon lime juice

- 1 teaspoon honey or maple syrup

- 1 garlic clove, minced

- 1/2 teaspoon grated ginger

- 1/4 teaspoon crushed red pepper flakes (optional)

Instructions

1. **Mix the Ingredients:** In a small bowl, whisk together the almond butter, coconut milk, soy sauce, lime juice, honey, garlic, and ginger until smooth.

2. **Adjust Consistency:** If the sauce is too thick, add more coconut milk or water until you reach your desired consistency.

3. **Season and Serve:** Stir in the crushed red pepper flakes if you like a bit of heat. Serve immediately or store in the refrigerator.

Chef's Tips

- **Consistency:** This sauce can be thinned with additional coconut milk or water if you prefer a lighter sauce.

- **Sweetness:** Adjust the sweetness by adding more or less honey or maple syrup according to your taste.

Nutritional Information

Calories: 100 (per tablespoon) | Protein: 2g | Total Fat: 9g | Saturated Fat: 2g | Cholesterol: 0mg | Sodium: 100mg | Fiber: 1g

Serving

- **With Grilled Meats:** Use a dipping sauce for grilled chicken or beef skewers.

- **As a Salad Dressing:** Thin out with more coconut milk and use as a dressing for an Asian-inspired salad.

Blue Cheese Dressing with Full-Fat Yogurt

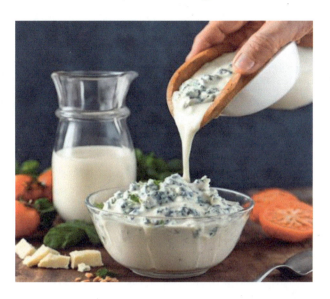

This rich and tangy blue cheese dressing has a creamy texture and is made with crumbled blue cheese and full-fat yogurt. It's perfect for drizzling over salads, as a veggie dip, or as a sauce for Buffalo wings.

Ingredients

- 1/2 cup full-fat Greek yogurt

- 1/4 cup mayonnaise

- 1/4 cup crumbled blue cheese

- 1 tablespoon lemon juice

- 1 garlic clove, minced

- 1 teaspoon Dijon mustard

- Salt and pepper to taste

Instructions

1. **Mix the Ingredients:** In a medium bowl, whisk together the Greek yogurt, mayonnaise, lemon juice, garlic, and Dijon mustard.

2. **Add the Blue Cheese:** Fold in the crumbled blue cheese, mixing until well combined.

3. **Season and Serve:** Season with salt and pepper to taste. Serve immediately or refrigerate until ready to use.

Chef's Tips

- **Texture:** Leave some larger pieces of blue cheese for a chunkier dressing. Blend the dressing in a food processor for a smoother consistency.

- **Storage:** Store in an airtight container in the refrigerator for up to a week.

Nutritional Information

Calories: 80 (per tablespoon) | Protein: 2g | Total Fat: 8g | Saturated Fat: 3g | Cholesterol: 10mg | Sodium: 150mg | Fiber: 0g

Serving

- **With Salads:** Drizzle over a wedge salad or use as a dressing for a Cobb salad.

- **As a Dip:** Serve for Buffalo wings, celery, or carrot sticks.

Spicy Buffalo Sauce with Ghee

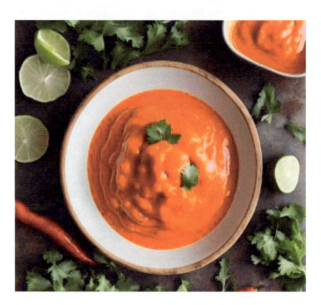

This spicy Buffalo sauce is made with rich ghee and hot sauce. It is bold and flavorful, perfect for coating chicken wings, drizzling over roasted vegetables, or using as a dip. The ghee adds a buttery richness that balances the heat.

Ingredients

- 1/2 cup hot sauce (such as Frank's RedHot)

- 1/4 cup ghee, melted

- 1 tablespoon apple cider vinegar

- 1/2 teaspoon garlic powder

- 1/4 teaspoon cayenne pepper (optional, for extra heat)

- Salt to taste

Instructions

1. **Combine Ingredients:** In a small saucepan, combine the hot sauce, melted ghee, apple cider vinegar, garlic powder, and cayenne pepper (if using).

2. **Heat the Sauce:** Place the saucepan over low heat and whisk the ingredients together until well combined and heated through.

3. **Season and Serve:** Taste and add salt if needed. Remove from heat and serve immediately, or keep warm until ready to use.

Chef's Tips

- **Adjusting Heat:** Reduce the hot sauce or omit the cayenne pepper for a milder sauce. For extra heat, add more cayenne's or a dash of Tabasco.

- **Storage:** Leftover sauce can be stored in an airtight container in the refrigerator for up to a week Reheat gently before use.

Nutritional Information

Calories: 80 (per tablespoon) | Protein: 0g | Total Fat: 9g | Saturated Fat: 5g | Cholesterol: 20mg | Sodium: 290mg | Fiber: 0g

Serving

- **With Wings:** Toss with chicken wings for classic Buffalo wings.

- **With Veggies:** Drizzle over roasted cauliflower or use it as a dipping sauce for celery sticks.

Tomato Basil Marinara with Olive Oil

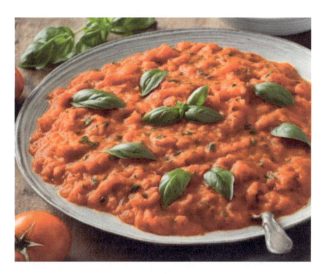

This homemade tomato basil marinara sauce is rich, flavorful, and made with simple ingredients. Olive oil adds depth and smoothness, while fresh basil and garlic bring out the tomatoes' natural sweetness. It's perfect for pasta, pizzas or as a base for other Italian dishes.

Ingredients

- 2 tablespoons extra virgin olive oil

- 4 garlic cloves, minced

- 1 can (28 ounces) crushed tomatoes

- 1/4 cup tomato paste

- 1/2 teaspoon dried oregano

- 1/2 teaspoon red pepper flakes (optional)

- 1/4 cup fresh basil leaves, chopped

- Salt and pepper to taste

Instructions

1. **Cook the Garlic:** Heat the olive oil in a large saucepan over medium heat. Add the

minced garlic and cook until fragrant, about 1 minute.

2. **Add Tomatoes and Seasonings:** Stir in the crushed tomatoes, tomato paste, oregano, and red pepper flakes. Bring to a simmer, then reduce heat to low and cook for 20-30 minutes, stirring occasionally.

3. **To finish the Sauce,** Stir in the chopped fresh basil and season with salt and pepper to taste. Simmer for an additional 5 minutes.

4. **Serve:** Serve the sauce immediately over pasta or use it as needed in other recipes.

Chef's Tips

- **Fresh vs. Canned:** Use fresh, ripe tomatoes instead of canned for a fresher taste. Blanch and peel them before cooking.

- **Blending:** Blend the marinara with an immersion blender after cooking for a smoother sauce.

Nutritional Information

Calories: 60 (per 1/2 cup) | Protein: 1g | Total Fat: 4g | Saturated Fat: 0.5g | Cholesterol: 0mg | Sodium: 300mg | Fiber: 2g

Serving

- **With Pasta:** Toss with your favorite pasta or use as a base for lasagna.

- **As a Pizza Sauce:** Spread over pizza dough before adding toppings and baking.

Coconut Curry Sauce

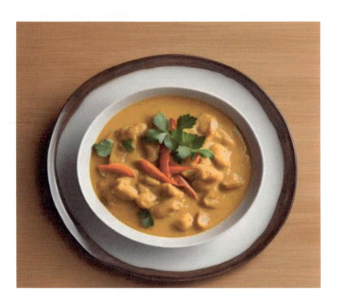

This coconut curry sauce is rich, creamy, and full of aromatic spices. It's versatile enough for vegetables, meats, and tofu. Made with coconut milk and a blend of curry spices, it is perfect for creating flavorful curries or as a dipping sauce.

Ingredients

- 1 can (14 ounces) coconut milk

- 1 tablespoon coconut oil

- 1 onion, finely chopped

- 3 garlic cloves, minced

- 1 tablespoon fresh ginger, minced

- 2 tablespoons curry powder

- 1 teaspoon ground turmeric

- 1/2 teaspoon ground cumin

- 1/2 teaspoon ground coriander

- 1/4 teaspoon cayenne pepper (optional)

- 1 tablespoon lime juice

- Salt to taste

Instructions

1. **Cook the Aromatics:** Heat the coconut oil in a medium saucepan over medium heat. Add the chopped onion, garlic, ginger, and sauté until the onion is soft and translucent.

2. **Add the Spices:** Stir in the curry powder, turmeric, cumin, coriander, and cayenne pepper (if using). Cook for 1-2 minutes until the spices are fragrant.

3. **Add Coconut Milk:** Pour in the coconut milk, stirring to combine with the spices. Bring the sauce to a simmer and cook for 10-15 minutes, stirring occasionally.

4. **To finish the Sauce,** Stir in the lime juice and season with salt to taste. Remove from heat and serve.

Chef's Tips

- **Spice Level:** Adjust the amount of cayenne pepper to control the sauce's heat. For a milder sauce, omit the cayenne altogether.

- **Storage:** Store in an airtight container in the refrigerator for up to 5 days. Reheat gently before serving.

Nutritional Information

Calories: 150 (per 1/4 cup) | Protein: 1g | Total Fat: 14g | Saturated Fat: 12g | Cholesterol: 0mg | Sodium: 200mg | Fiber: 1g

Serving

- **With Rice:** Serve over steamed jasmine rice or basmati rice.

- **With Grilled Meats:** Use as a sauce for grilled chicken, shrimp, or tofu.

Creamy Garlic Parmesan Sauce

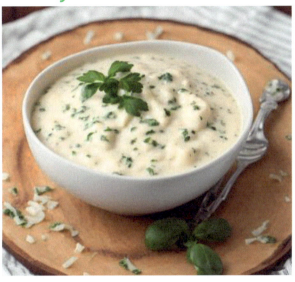

This creamy garlic Parmesan sauce is rich and velvety, made with garlic, Parmesan cheese, and a hint of cream. It's perfect for pasta, drizzling over roasted vegetables, or as a sauce for chicken or seafood.

Ingredients

- 2 tablespoons butter

- 4 garlic cloves, minced

- 1 cup heavy cream

- 1/2 cup grated Parmesan cheese

- 1/4 teaspoon ground black pepper

- Salt to taste

- Fresh parsley, chopped (optional, for garnish)

Instructions

1. **Cook the Garlic:** Melt the butter in a medium saucepan over medium heat. Add

the minced garlic and cook for 1-2 minutes, until fragrant and lightly golden.

2. **Add the Cream:** Stir in the heavy cream and bring the mixture to a simmer. Cook for 5-7 minutes, stirring occasionally, until the sauce thickens.

3. **Add the Parmesan:** Stir in the grated cheese until thoroughly melted and the sauce is smooth—season with black pepper and salt to taste.

4. **Serve:** Remove from heat and serve immediately, garnished with chopped parsley if desired.

Chef's Tips

- **Cheese Quality:** Use freshly grated Parmesan cheese for the best flavor and texture.

- **Thickening:** If the sauce is too thin, let it simmer until it reaches your desired consistency.

Nutritional Information

Calories: 200 (per 1/4 cup) | Protein: 4g | Total Fat: 20g | Saturated Fat: 12g | Cholesterol: 60mg | Sodium: 250mg | Fiber: 0g

Serving

- **With Pasta:** Toss with fettuccine or penne for a rich, creamy pasta dish.

- **With Vegetables:** Drizzle over roasted broccoli, cauliflower, or asparagus.

Conclusion

Recap of Key Principles

As we conclude this journey through healthier cooking and eating, we must reflect on the principles that have guided us throughout this book. We've explored the power of natural, unprocessed ingredients, the benefits of traditional fats over modern, highly processed oils, and the joy of creating flavorful meals that nourish both body and soul. By embracing these principles, you've taken a significant step toward a healthier lifestyle that prioritizes real food and the wisdom of traditional cooking.

Encouragement to Continue the Journey

Your journey doesn't end here it's just beginning. Every recipe you've tried and every new ingredient you've embraced has brought you closer to a more vibrant, health-conscious way of living. Remember that change is a process, and each small step is a victory. Continue experimenting with the recipes, exploring new flavors, and sharing your culinary creations with friends and family. As you continue on this path, you'll find that cooking with natural, wholesome ingredients becomes second nature, and the benefits will continue to unfold in your daily life.

Your Feedback Matters

If you've enjoyed this book and found it helpful, please leave a review. Your feedback helps other readers discover this resource and allows me to continue improving and providing valuable content. Sharing your thoughts and experiences with the recipes and principles in this book can inspire others to embark on their journey toward better health. Thank you for joining me on this culinary adventure I hope it brings you many delicious and healthful meals in the future.

Bonus

Week 1

Day 1

- **Breakfast:** Classic Scrambled Eggs with Grass-Fed Butter
- **Lunch:** Mediterranean Chicken Salad with Olive Oil Dressing
- **Dinner:** Garlic Butter Steak with Roasted Vegetables
- **Snack:** Baked Kale Chips with Sea Salt

Day 2

- **Breakfast:** Coconut Flour Pancakes with Pure Maple Syrup
- **Lunch:** Wild-caught tuna Salad with Avocado Oil Mayo
- **Dinner:** Baked Salmon with Lemon Herb Ghee Sauce
- **Snack:** Guacamole with Homemade Almond Flour Chips

Day 3

- **Breakfast:** Full-Fat Greek Yogurt with Berries and Honey
- **Lunch:** Zucchini Noodles with Pesto and Chicken
- **Dinner:** Chicken Thighs in Coconut Milk Curry

- **Snack:** Spicy Roasted Chickpeas in Olive Oil

Day 4

- **Breakfast:** Avocado and Poached Egg Toast on Sourdough
- **Lunch:** Cobb Salad with Olive Oil and Red Wine Vinaigrette
- **Dinner:** Pork Tenderloin with Mustard Cream Sauce
- **Snack:** Almond Butter Stuffed Dates

Day 5

- **Breakfast:** Almond Flour Waffles with Ghee
- **Lunch:** Spinach and Goat Cheese Stuffed Chicken Breast
- **Dinner:** Grilled Shrimp and Avocado Salad
- **Snack:** Coconut Macaroons with Dark Chocolate Drizzle

Day 6

- **Breakfast:** Chia Seed Pudding with Coconut Milk
- **Lunch:** Roasted Vegetable Quinoa Bowl with Tahini Dressing
- **Dinner:** Herb-crusted roast Beef with Garlic Butter
- **Snack:** Cream Cheese and Smoked Salmon Bites

Day 7

- **Breakfast:** Smoked Salmon and Cream Cheese Omelette

- **Lunch:** Turkey Lettuce Wraps with Avocado Cream

- **Dinner:** Chicken Marsala with Mushroom Sauce

- **Snack:** Cucumber Slices with Cream Cheese and Herbs

Week 2

Day 8

- **Breakfast:** Spinach and Feta Frittata

- **Lunch:** Baked Cod with Lemon Butter Sauce

- **Dinner:** Braised Short Ribs with Red Wine and Vegetables

- **Snack:** Deviled Ham Spread with Almond Crackers

Day 9

- **Breakfast:** Bulletproof Coffee with MCT Oil

- **Lunch:** Eggplant Parmesan with Almond Flour

- **Dinner:** Lamb Chops with Mint Yogurt Sauce

- **Snack:** Guacamole with Fresh Veggies

Day 10

- **Breakfast:** Bacon and Egg Muffins

- **Lunch:** Pulled Pork Lettuce Wraps with Salsa Verde

- **Dinner:** Shrimp Scampi with Zoodles

- **Snack:** Baked Kale Chips with Sea Salt

Day 11

- **Breakfast:** Sweet Potato Hash with Eggs and Avocado Oil

- **Lunch:** Chicken Caesar Salad with Homemade Dressing

- **Dinner:** Pork Tenderloin with Mustard Cream Sauce

- **Snack:** Bacon-Wrapped Jalapeño Poppers

Day 12

- **Breakfast:** Keto-Friendly Smoothie with Coconut Milk

- **Lunch:** Grilled Chicken with Avocado Salsa

- **Dinner:** Beef Stroganoff with Creamy Coconut Milk Sauce

- **Snack:** Marinated Artichokes and Olives

Day 13

- **Breakfast:** Grain-Free Granola with Nuts and Seeds

- **Lunch:** Greek Salad with Feta and Kalamata Olives

- **Dinner:** Spaghetti Squash Bolognese

- **Snack:** Almond Butter Stuffed Dates

Day 14

- **Breakfast:** Shakshuka with Olive Oil

- **Lunch:** Cauliflower Rice stir-fried with Coconut Aminos

- **Dinner:** Chicken Thighs in Coconut Milk Curry

- **Snack:** Coconut Macaroons with Dark Chocolate Drizzle

Week 3

- **Breakfast:** Coconut Flour Breakfast Biscuits

- **Lunch:** Mediterranean Chicken Salad with Olive Oil Dressing

- **Dinner:** Garlic Butter Steak with Roasted Vegetables

- **Snack:** Spicy Roasted Chickpeas in Olive Oil

Day 16

- **Breakfast:** Classic Scrambled Eggs with Grass-Fed Butter

- **Lunch:** Wild-caught tuna Salad with Avocado Oil Mayo

- **Dinner:** Baked Salmon with Lemon Herb Ghee Sauce

- **Snack:** Deviled Ham Spread with Almond Crackers

Day 17

- **Breakfast:** Full-fat Greek Yogurt with Berries and Honey

- **Lunch:** Zucchini Noodles with Pesto and Chicken

- **Dinner:** Herb-crusted roast Beef with Garlic Butter

- **Snack:** Cream Cheese and Smoked Salmon Bites

Day 18

- **Breakfast:** Avocado and Poached Egg Toast on Sourdough

- **Lunch:** Cobb Salad with Olive Oil and Red Wine Vinaigrette

- **Dinner:** Chicken Marsala with Mushroom Sauce

- **Snack:** Baked Kale Chips with Sea Salt

Day 19

- **Breakfast:** Almond Flour Waffles with Ghee

- **Lunch:** Spinach and Goat Cheese Stuffed Chicken Breast

- **Dinner:** Grilled Shrimp and Avocado Salad

- **Snack:** Guacamole with Fresh Veggies

Day 20

- **Breakfast:** Chia Seed Pudding with Coconut Milk

- **Lunch:** Roasted Vegetable Quinoa Bowl with Tahini Dressing

- **Dinner:** Lamb Chops with Mint Yogurt Sauce

- **Snack:** Bacon-Wrapped Jalapeño Poppers

Day 21

- **Breakfast:** Smoked Salmon and Cream Cheese Omelette

- **Lunch:** Turkey Lettuce Wraps with Avocado Cream

- **Dinner:** Shrimp Scampi with Zoodles

- **Snack:** Almond Butter Stuffed Dates

Week 4

Day 22

- **Breakfast:** Spinach and Feta Frittata

- **Lunch:** Baked Cod with Lemon Butter Sauce

- **Dinner:** Braised Short Ribs with Red Wine and Vegetables

- **Snack:** Cucumber Slices with Cream Cheese and Herbs

Day 23

- **Breakfast:** Bulletproof Coffee with MCT Oil

- **Lunch:** Eggplant Parmesan with Almond Flour

- **Dinner:** Beef Stroganoff with Creamy Coconut Milk Sauce

- **Snack:** Deviled Ham Spread with Almond Crackers

Day 24

- **Breakfast:** Bacon and Egg Muffins

- **Lunch:** Pulled Pork Lettuce Wraps with Salsa Verde

- **Dinner:** Chicken Thighs in Coconut Milk Curry

- **Snack:** Spicy Roasted Chickpeas in Olive Oil

Day 25

- **Breakfast:** Sweet Potato Hash with Eggs and Avocado Oil

- **Lunch:** Chicken Caesar Salad with Homemade Dressing

- **Dinner:** Lamb Chops with Mint Yogurt Sauce

- **Snack:** Guacamole with Homemade Almond Flour Chips

Day 26

- **Breakfast:** Keto-Friendly Smoothie with Coconut Milk

- **Lunch:** Grilled Chicken with Avocado Salsa

- **Dinner:** Pork Tenderloin with Mustard Cream Sauce

- **Snack:** Coconut Macaroons with Dark Chocolate Drizzle

Day 27

- **Breakfast:** Grain-Free Granola with Nuts and Seeds

- **Lunch:** Greek Salad with Feta and Kalamata Olives

- **Dinner:** Shrimp Scampi with Zoodles

- **Snack:** Almond Butter Stuffed Dates

Day 28

- **Breakfast:** Shakshuka with Olive Oil

- **Lunch:** Cauliflower Rice stir-fried with Coconut Aminos

- **Dinner:** Chicken Marsala with Mushroom Sauce

- **Snack:** Marinated Artichokes and Olives

Week 5

Day 29

- **Breakfast:** Coconut Flour Breakfast Biscuits

- **Lunch:** Mediterranean Chicken Salad with Olive Oil Dressing

- **Dinner:** Garlic Butter Steak with Roasted Vegetables

- **Snack:** Baked Kale Chips with Sea Salt

Day 30

- **Breakfast:** Classic Scrambled Eggs with Grass-Fed Butter

- **Lunch:** Wild-caught tuna Salad with Avocado Oil Mayo

- **Dinner:** Baked Salmon with Lemon Herb Ghee Sauce

- **Snack:** Cream Cheese and Smoked Salmon Bites

Appendix

Glossary of Terms

Avocado Oil is healthy, nutrient-rich oil made from the flesh of avocados. Its high smoke point makes it ideal for cooking and frying.

Coconut Milk: A creamy liquid extracted from the grated pulp of mature coconuts. It is a common ingredient in many Southeast Asian dishes and is often used as a dairy-free alternative in cooking.

Ghee: Clarified butter simmered to remove milk solids, resulting in a rich, nutty flavor. Ghee is commonly used in Indian cuisine and is favored for its high smoke point and health benefits.

Grass-Fed Butter: Butter made from the milk of cows fed a diet primarily consisting of grass. It is richer in omega-3 fatty acids and vitamins A and E compared to conventional butter.

Tahini: A paste made from ground sesame seeds, commonly used in Middle Eastern cuisine. It is a crucial ingredient in hummus and dressings.

Zoodles: A popular low-carb alternative to pasta, made by spiralizing zucchini into noodle-like strands.

Bocconcini: Small balls of fresh mozzarella cheese, often used in salads and appetizers like Caprese skewers.

Bulletproof Coffee: A high-calorie coffee drink made with butter and MCT oil, popularized by the ketogenic diet for its energy-boosting properties.

Chipotle Pepper: A smoked, dried jalapeño pepper, often found canned in adobo sauce. It adds a smoky, spicy flavor to dishes.

Nutritional Yeast: A deactivated yeast often used as a vegan cheese substitute. It has a nutty, cheesy flavor and is rich in B vitamins.

Conversion Charts

Common Volume Measurements

- 1 teaspoon (tsp) = 5 milliliters (ml)

- 1 tablespoon (tbsp) = 3 teaspoons (tsp) = 15 milliliters (ml)

- 1/4 cup = 4 tablespoons (tbsp) = 60 milliliters (ml)

- 1/3 cup = 5 tablespoons + 1 teaspoon = 80 milliliters (ml)

- 1/2 cup = 8 tablespoons (tbsp) = 120 milliliters (ml)

- 1 cup = 16 tablespoons (tbsp) = 240 milliliters (ml)

Common Weight Measurements

- 1 ounce (oz) = 28 grams (g)

- 1 pound (lb) = 16 ounces (oz) = 454 grams (g)

Oven Temperature Conversions

- 250°F = 120°C (very slow)

- 300°F = 150°C (slow)

- 350°F = 180°C (moderate)

- 400°F = 200°C (moderately hot)

- 450°F = 230°C (hot)

Recommended Suppliers for Quality Fats and Ingredients

1. US Wellness Meats

- **Products:** Grass-fed butter, ghee, and other grass-fed animal products.
- **Description:** A trusted source for high-quality, grass-fed, pasture-raised meats, dairy, and oils.

2. Thrive Market

- **Products:** Organic coconut milk, avocado oil, olive oil, and pantry staples.
- **Description:** An online marketplace offering natural and organic products at discounted prices.

3. Primal Kitchen

- **Products:** Avocado oil mayonnaise, dressings, and sauces.
- **Description:** A brand focused on healthy fats and clean ingredients, ideal for paleo and keto lifestyles.

4. Vital Choice

- **Products:** Wild-caught seafood, olive oil, and coconut products.
- **Description:** Specializes in sustainable, wild-caught seafood and other natural foods.

5. Azure Standard

- **Products:** Organic nuts, seeds, grains, and other bulk ingredients.
- **Description:** A bulk and natural foods supplier offering a wide range of organic products.

Index of Recipes

Breakfast

Lunch

- Mediterranean Chicken Salad with Olive Oil Dressing - Day 1, 15, 29
- Wild-Caught Tuna Salad with Avocado Oil Mayo - Day 2, 16, 30
- Zucchini Noodles with Pesto and Chicken - Day 3, 17
- Cobb Salad with Olive Oil and Red Wine Vinaigrette - Day 4, 18
- Spinach and Goat Cheese Stuffed Chicken Breast - Day 5, 19
- Roasted Vegetable Quinoa Bowl with Tahini Dressing - Day 6, 20
- Turkey Lettuce Wraps with Avocado Cream - Day 7, 21
- Baked Cod with Lemon Butter Sauce - Day 8, 22
- Eggplant Parmesan with Almond Flour - Day 9, 23
- Pulled Pork Lettuce Wraps with Salsa Verde - Day 10, 24
- Chicken Caesar Salad with Homemade Dressing - Day 11, 25
- Grilled Chicken with Avocado Salsa - Day 12, 26
- Greek Salad with Feta and Kalamata Olives - Day 13, 27
- Cauliflower Rice Stir-Fry with Coconut Aminos - Day 14, 28

Dinner

- Garlic Butter Steak with Roasted Vegetables - Day 1, 15, 29
- Baked Salmon with Lemon Herb Ghee Sauce - Day 2, 16, 30
- Chicken Thighs in Coconut Milk Curry - Day 3, 20, 24, 28
- Pork Tenderloin with Mustard Cream Sauce - Day 4, 11, 26
- Grilled Shrimp and Avocado Salad - Day 5, 19
- Herb-Crusted Roast Beef with Garlic Butter - Day 6, 17
- Chicken Marsala with Mushroom Sauce - Day 7, 18, 28
- Braised Short Ribs with Red Wine and Vegetables - Day 8, 22
- Lamb Chops with Mint Yogurt Sauce - Day 9, 20, 25
- Shrimp Scampi with Zoodles - Day 10, 21, 27
- Beef Stroganoff with Creamy Coconut Milk Sauce - Day 12, 23
- Spaghetti Squash Bolognese - Day 13
- Chicken Thighs in Coconut Milk Curry - Day 14, 28

Snacks and Appetizers

- Baked Kale Chips with Sea Salt - Day 1, 10, 18, 29
- Guacamole with Homemade Almond Flour Chips - Day 2, 25

- Spicy Roasted Chickpeas in Olive Oil - Day 3, 10, 15, 24

- Almond Butter Stuffed Dates - Day 4, 13, 21, 27

- Coconut Macaroons with Dark Chocolate Drizzle - Day 5, 14, 26

- Cream Cheese and Smoked Salmon Bites - Day 6, 17, 30

- Bacon-Wrapped Jalapeño Poppers - Day 11, 20

- Deviled Ham Spread with Almond Crackers - Day 8, 16, 23

- Cucumber Slices with Cream Cheese and Herbs - Day 7, 22

- Marinated Artichokes and Olives - Day 12, 28

Made in United States
Troutdale, OR
03/18/2025

29865610R00058